UNDERSTANDING THE NURSING PROCESS

Pergamon Titles of Related Interest

UNDERSTANDING THE NURSING PROCESS

Fundamentals of Care Planning

Fourth Edition

Leslie D. Atkinson, R.N., M.S.
Nursing Program
Normandale Community College
Bloomington, Minnesota

and

Mary Ellen Murray, R.N., M.S.
Doctoral Student in Nursing
University of Michigan
Ann Arbor, Michigan

Illustrated by Mark Atkinson

PERGAMON PRESS
Member of Maxwell Macmillan Pergamon Publishing Corporation
New York • Oxford • Beijing • Frankfurt
São Paulo • Sydney • Tokyo • Toronto

Pergamon Press Offices:

U.S.A.	Pergamon Press, Inc., Maxwell House, Fairview Park, Elmsford, New York 10523, U.S.A.
U.K.	Pergamon Press plc, Headington Hill Hall, Oxford OX3 OBW, England
PEOPLE'S REPUBLIC OF CHINA	Pergamon Press, 0909 China World Tower, No. 1, Jian Guo Men Wai Avenue, Beijing 100004, People's Republic of China
FEDERAL REPUBLIC OF GERMANY	Pergamon Press GmbH, Hammerweg 6, D-6242 Kronberg, Federal Republic of Germany
BRAZIL	Pergamon Editora Ltda, Rua Eca de Querios, 346, CEP 04011, Paraiso, São Paulo, Brazil
AUSTRALIA	Pergamon Press Australia Pty Ltd., P.O. Box 544, Potts Point, N.S.W. 2011, Australia
JAPAN	Pergamon Press, 8th Floor, Matsuoka Central Building, 1-7-1 Nishishinjuku, Shinjuku-ku, Tokyo 160, Japan
CANADA	Pergamon Press Canada Ltd., Suite No. 271, 253 College Street, Toronto, Ontario, Canada M5T 1R5

Library of Congress Cataloging in Publication Data

Atkinson, Leslie D.
    Understanding the nursing process: fundamentals of care planning
    / by Leslie D. Atkinson and Mary Ellen Murray: illustrated by Mark
Atkinson.—4th ed.
      p. cm.
    Includes bibliographical references.
    ISBN 0-08-040299-2 (soft)
    1. Nursing. 2. Diagnosis. I. Murray, Mary Ellen. II. Title.
    [DNLM: 1. Nursing Process. WY 100 A876u]
RT41.A82   1990
610.73—dc20
DNLM/DLC   89-71116
for Library of Congress   CIP

Printing: 1 2 3 4 5 6 7 8 9   Year: 0 1 2 3 4 5 6 7 8 9

Printed in the United States of America

Dedication
To Gary
To Peter

Preface to the Fourth Edition

Since the publication of the first edition of *Understanding the Nursing Process,* in 1980, we have seen an increasing necessity and responsibility for students to enter the profession of nursing with a consistent and organized framework for approaching patient care. This framework or way of "thinking as a nurse" is best introduced and developed very early in the student's educational program, regardless of its length. We believe the nursing process and the concept of care planning should be introduced in the first nursing course, even though the student may not yet have the knowledge to understand complex treatments and plans of care. Students continue to ask for a practical, understandable, fundamentals text on the nursing process matched to their nursing knowledge level as they begin to have experiences in the clinical setting. This text is designed to introduce the process, to motivate the student to use the process, and to help the student begin to initiate problem-solving thinking into all aspects of patient care. It is our belief that as the student advances through nursing courses, more advanced, theoretical aspects of problem-solving and clinical decision making need to be presented. In later nursing courses, the student's knowledge base and clinical experience has grown to permit understanding and integration of these concepts. Because this text is written for a student entering nursing education, terminology and nursing/medical interventions are kept simple and theoretical discussions of nursing, nursing process, and conceptual models for nursing are presented only in the very practical sense of application to fundamental patient care planning situations.

We continue to see trends within health care that make the nursing process an essential tool in all types of delivery systems:

1. Decreasing length of stay in the hospital. Patients are being discharged in less and less time because of limits imposed by health insurance payments. Same-day surgery is increasingly used as a cost effective alternative to hospitalization further limiting the time the professional nurse has to spend with an individual patient. Assessment, diagnosis, and planning become even more crucial as families and home health agencies provide care previously done by nurses in the hospital.

2. Expansion of home health care. Various types of health care personnel such as home health aides, LPNs, and RNs are providing care to people in their homes to facilitate early hospital discharge or to enable people to remain in their own homes rather than being admitted to nursing homes. Without a thorough assessment, accurate diagnoses, and effective plans developed by the professional nurse, the care may be less than optimal. The health care provider may have inadequate guidelines for health promotion and maintenance in the home care setting.

3. Further clarification of nursing diagnoses and refinement of a taxonomy of nursing diagnoses by the North American Nursing Diagnosis Association (NANDA) at the Eighth Conference. The addition of major defining characteristics which must be present to diagnose a particular problem will affect application in both the educational and clinical setting.

4. Increased clinical use of standardized care plans based on nursing diagnoses developed by NANDA to replace the handwritten, individually developed care plans. Individualizing a preprinted or computer generated care plan for a particular diagnostic category is a different level clinical skill than creation of a care plan. We have incorporated several examples of how standardized care plans can be individualized in addition to the traditional form. We see individualization of these standard care plans becoming the norm in the clinical setting replacing the traditional nurse generated plan for each patient.

5. Increasing scope of independent nursing interventions.

6. Increasing acuity levels of hospitalized patients.

7. Increasing legal accountability of nurses for nursing practice.

8. Hospital accreditation standards requiring an RN to develop the plan of nursing care using the nursing process and documenting the plan and the outcomes in the chart.

9. Utilization of the registered nurse licensing examination based on the nursing process steps of: assessing, analyzing, planning, implementing, evaluating.

10. Utilization of the concept of collaborative problems between nurse and physician. These problems are different from nursing diagnoses, in that nursing is not primarily responsible for planning the definitive treatment. Assessment of the problem and the plan of care usually involves both collaborative and independent nursing interventions. The nursing process is an essential component of this collaborative role, and complements the traditional view of the nursing process as involving patient problems and treatments solely within the scope of nursing practice.

As in the third edition, the fourth edition will emphasize a practical approach to utilizing the nursing process and developing patient care plans. Other features of the fourth edition include:

—inclusion of standardized care plans for several NANDA diagnostic groups, individualized in different ways based on different patient examples.

—addition of a separate chapter on diagnosis to reflect the increasing emphasis on this process.

—inclusion of vignettes to exemplify points within the text.

—inclusion of a pocketbook of nursing diagnoses from the Eighth NANDA Conference which includes definitions and defining characteristics for quick reference by students in the clinical setting.

—utilization of three different frameworks for nursing assessment of the client in care plan examples: basic needs based on work by Maslow, functional health patterns based on work by Gordon (1982), and human response patterns based on NANDA's taxonomy of nursing diagnoses (1989).

We wish to express our appreciation to the nurse educators who have given us encouragement and constructive criticism from our first three editions and to NANDA for their continued development and clarification of nursing diagnoses. We wish to thank our students who continually force us to apply our theoretical concepts to actual patient care settings in an efficient and effective way and who question traditional ways of doing things until we hear them and critically examine what and how we teach. We wish to acknowledge the contributions of Tom Olson, RN, MSN, PhD Candidate, for his initial work with care plan #2 in Appendix A and Mark Atkinson for his cartoon art.

—LDA
—MEM

Contents

Chapter 3:   Planning   51

The Nursing Process

NURSING: WHAT IS IT?

Nursing has been described in many different ways by many different leaders and theorists in nursing. What is special about nursing? What service do we provide to our patients that no other health care professional provides? In 1980 the American Nurses' Association, which is the professional organization for nurses in the United States, developed a definition that is current and basic to describe the scope of nursing practice.

> Nursing is the diagnosis and treatment of human responses to actual or potential health problems. (A.N.A., "Nursing—A Social Policy Statement," 1980)

This means, for example, that nursing is not responsible for diagnosing and treating cancer; the physician does this. Nursing is primarily responsible for diagnosing and treating a patient's *response* to the cancer and medical treatment, such as inadequate nutrition, nausea, altered self-esteem, anxiety, and pain. Nursing is involved in aspects of the medical treatment as when giving a patient prescribed medication or treatments, but the primary focus of nursing is the individual's response to health-related problems.

THE NURSING PROCESS: WHAT IS IT?

The nursing process is a problem-solving framework for planning and delivering nursing care to patients and their families.

The nursing process is:

- a way of thinking as a nurse
- a framework of interrelated activities resulting in competent nursing care
- dynamic and cyclical in nature, requiring repeated review
- a scientific, problem-oriented approach to patient care

The nursing process is divided into five steps:

1. Assessment
        Let me have a look at that.
        Tell me about it.
2. Diagnosis
        What is the problem?
        What is the cause?
        How do I know it?
3. Planning
        What are we going to do about it?
        What is the best strategy?
        What do we want to happen?
4. Implementation
        Move into action.
        Carry out the plan.
        Do it, to it!
5. Evaluation
        Did it work? Why didn't it work?
        Did we end up where we wanted to?
        Are we done or is there more? What's the problem?

During this process, a written nursing care plan is developed. While the above descriptions are an oversimplification, every nurse already has had much practice in using similar problem-solving techniques, even though the terms of the nursing process itself may be unfamiliar. Consider a high-school chemistry class. Students are asked to observe and examine the properties of different chemicals, and to perform a series of planned experiments utilizing those substances. The student then records and evaluates the results. Hopefully, the student, through the use of this scientific problem-solving process, has discovered the solution to the problem of how certain chemicals react. These steps are essentially the same as those utilized in the nursing process. More familiar is the case of the father who observes the chaos of his 7-year-old's bedroom. After giving the scene an eyeball ASSESSMENT, and palpating the bedcovers for any sign of life, he DIAGNOSES the problem, "This room is an absolute mess!" He then sets forth a PLAN of action. He chooses a goal, "That child isn't going out to play until all his toys are put away." He recruits his son to IMPLE-MENT the clean-up, and finally EVALUATES the results. These examples point out that a problem-solving process is not only important to the sciences but is also an integral activity of daily living. Similarly, the applied science of nursing utilizes a logical, systematic problem-solving process to deliver its services. This is called the nursing process. Patients' written care plans are based on application of the nursing process. These care plans serve as a guide for patient care.

WHY IS THE NURSING PROCESS IMPORTANT?

When used as a tool in nursing practice, the nursing process can help ensure quality patient care. Without this systematic way of approaching patient care, omissions and duplications begin to occur. A nursing care plan helps to reduce these problems when it is used as a guide in providing care for a particular patient. Just as a physician formulates medical care plans in treating patients' diseases to ensure consistent, responsible medical management, a nurse utilizes the nursing process to create care plans to ensure consistent and responsible nursing management of patients' problems.

While the primary benefit of utilizing the nursing process is improved patient care, there are also definite advantages for the individual nurse who becomes skilled in the use of this tool. Consider the following advantages for the nurse (and the student):

1. **Graduation from an Accredited School of Nursing.** All levels of nursing programs (diploma, associate degree, and baccalaureate) require students to have a basic competency in the use of the nursing process upon graduation.
2. **Confidence.** Care plans resulting from the nursing process let the student or the staff nurse know specifically what problem the patient has, what goals are important for the patient, and how and when they might best be accomplished.
3. **Job Satisfaction.** Good care plans can save time, energy, and the frustration that is generated by trial-and-error nursing from staff members and students whose efforts remain uncoordinated. Coordinating a patient's nursing care through a care plan greatly increases the chances of achieving a successful resolution of health

problems. The nurse and student should feel a real sense of accomplishment and professional pride when goals in a care plan are met.

4. **Professional Growth.** Care plans provide an opportunity to share knowledge and experience. Collaboration with colleagues in formulating a nursing care plan will add to an inexperienced nurse's clinical skills. Later, during the process of evaluation, the nurse or student receives the feedback necessary to decide how effective the nursing care plan was in dealing with the patient's problems. If the plan worked well, the nurse may use a similar approach in the future. If it failed, the nurse can explore possible reasons for the undesirable results with the patient, other staff, other students, an instructor, or a clinical nurse specialist.

5. **Aid in Staff Assignments.** Care plans assist charge nurses, team leaders, and nursing instructors in making the most appropriate patient assignments by showing the degree of complexity involved in an individual patient's care plan. Could an aide follow the care plan and provide good care, or is a professional nurse required? Could students work with this patient or is the plan of care beyond their knowledge and experience? What aspects of nursing care can be safely delegated?

6. **Employment in a Nationally Accredited Hospital.** Hospitals are approved by a national commission to help ensure that patients receive quality care. The following statement is taken directly from the accreditation manual for hospitals and is a requirement for accreditation. (JCAHO, *Accreditation Manual*, 1989).

    Standard IV
    Individualized, goal-directed nursing care is provided to patients through the use of the nursing process.

7. **Meeting Standards of Nursing Practice.** The American Nurses' Association has identified eight standards of nursing practice that are activities in the nursing process (A.N.A., *Standards of Nursing Practice*, 1973). See Table 1.

There are also advantages for the patient.

1. **Participation in Own Care.** If patients are able to help formulate their own care plans with the nurse, they gain a sense of their own ability to solve problems. When patients are active participants in their care, they are more likely to be committed to the goals in their care plans and thus achieve improved health.

2. **Continuity of Care.** The frustration of repeating the same infor-

Table 1 Standards of Nursing Practice

I. The collection of data about the health status of the client/patient is systematic and continuous. The data are accessible, communicated, and recorded.

II. Nursing diagnoses are derived from health status data.

III. The plan of nursing care includes goals derived from the nursing diagnoses.

IV. The plan of nursing care includes the priorities and the prescribed nursing approaches or measures to achieve the goals derived from the nursing diagnoses.

V. Nursing actions provide for client/patient participation in health promotion, maintenance, and restoration.

VI. Nursing actions assist the client/patient to maximize his or her health capabilities.

VII. The client's/patient's progress or lack of progress toward goal achievement is determined by the client/patient and the nurse.

VIII. The client's/patient's progress or lack of progress toward goal achievement directs reassessment, reordering of priorities, new goal setting, and revision of the plan of nursing care.

Reproduced with the permission of A.N.A. from *Standards of Nursing Practice*, A.N.A., 1973.

mation to each nurse caring for them is greatly reduced. Worries, concerns, and problems need not be communicated to each nurse to ensure that they are handled the way patients want them to be handled. The care plan communicates this information.

3. Improved Quality of Care. Use of the nursing process results in a thorough assessment of the patient at the time of admission. Problems are identified at this time by an RN, who then develops a plan of nursing care with the patient. This plan, developed by the nurse most familiar with the patient, serves as a guide for other nurses, assistants, and students to follow in providing 24-hour care to the patient. Continuous evaluation and review of the plan of care assures a level of care that will better meet changing individual needs. This evaluation is a key part of the nursing process and a patient's written care plan.

Giving nursing care without a care plan is like trying to cook a nameless entree without a recipe. To add to your troubles, you have to share the work for preparing this entree with three other cooks, all in the kitchen at different times. You can all cook, but a plan is needed to tell you what the entree is, how to prepare it, when to serve it, and how the three of you can coordinate your efforts to produce the best entree possible. Similarly, many nurses share in the care of a single patient throughout the 24-hour hospital day. Each nurse is capable of providing care, but a plan is needed to coordinate their efforts.

WHAT DOES IT LOOK LIKE?

When the nursing process is being utilized, you will find patients who report that they are receiving excellent nursing care by nurses who really understand their problems and are concerned about them as individuals. You will find an assessment form in the patient's chart indicating that the admitting RN took the time to discuss patient and family concerns and current health-related problems. The use of the nursing process will result in a care plan describing the problems and care for each patient. There are many forms the nursing care plan may take. It may be handwritten on a form designed by the institution or it may be a computerized print out that the nurse has adapted for the needs of a specific patient. But, whatever format it takes, the plan will include the five essential elements of care: assessment, diagnoses, goals, nursing interventions, and evaluations.

CHAPTER 1

Assessment

I. The collection of data about the health status of the client/patient is systematic and continuous. The data are accessible, communicated, and recorded. (Standards of Nursing Practice, American Nurses' Association, 1973)

Assessment (data collection) is both the initial step in the nursing process and an ongoing component of every other step in the process. Assessment is the process of collecting data for the purpose of identifying actual or potential patient health problems which the professional nurse is licensed to treat. Assessment is part of each activity the nurse does for and with the patient. The initial nursing assessment is the basis of the patient care plan and later assessments contribute to revisions and updates in the plan as the patient's condition changes. All individuals are constantly using their five senses to assess changes in their environment to make necessary changes and adapt to it. One person may note the cold temperature and dress more warmly while a second person is aware of a toothache and seeks dental care. Nurses too, are constantly seeking information about the patient through their five senses and processing it to identify changes in status and intervene appropriately.

Assessment (Data Collection) = Observation + Interview + Examination

---

DATA COLLECTION

Initially the beginning nursing student collects data on the individual patient, but families, groups, and communities can all be the focus of a nursing assessment by more advanced nurses. Because human beings are extraordinarily complex and because assessment is an ongoing process, there is the potential for the nurse to collect an overwhelming amount of data. It is unrealistic to think that the nurse will record every bit of information that could be obtained. One component of the skill of assessment is the ability of the nurse to collect *relevant* data. The nursing care plan will be only as good as the data that go into it. A saying used by computerniks nicely illustrates this point, "Garbage in, garbage out."

Data Collection Format

Beginning nursing students are often required to complete nursing data collection assignments. Often these assignments are very lengthy and time-consuming. The purpose of such an assignment is to assist the student in a comprehensive data review and to avoid errors of omission. After the student has demonstrated proficiency in this skill, an abbreviated data collection format similar to those used by staff nurses is recommended. Several examples of such forms will be used throughout this book.

Most hospitals or other health care institutions use a form to guide the collection of data when the nurse is admitting the patient. This form is usually labeled *Nursing Admission Assessment*. The structure of this form will vary with the institution. A structured form is used to avoid omitting

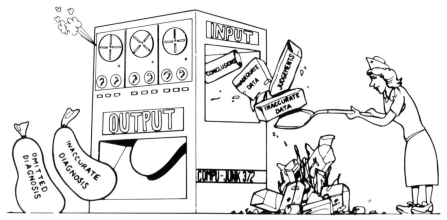

FIGURE 1–1.   Garbage in, garbage out.

data in important human response areas and to give the patient an opportunity to discuss problems or request information in these areas. For example, when nurses (students and staff) complete an admission assessment, they frequently avoid initiating any discussion of sexuality or sexual behavior either by skipping the item completely or by making the item "NA" which means "not applicable." Although this may enhance the student's comfort level at the time, it does not contribute to a comprehensive assessment of the patient. The nursing admission form includes this category thus identifying it as important and encouraging nurses to do more complete assessment even though there may initially be hesitancy or discomfort in asking questions in this area.

Maslow's Basic Need Framework. One assessment framework that is frequently used to guide the collection of data is based on the work of psychologist Abraham Maslow (1968), who postulated that all human beings have common basic needs that can be arranged in a hierarchical order (Table 1-1). Maslow further theorized that basic physical needs must be met to some degree before higher level needs can be met.

Table 1–1   Common Basic Human Needs

1. Physiological needs—needs that must be met, or at least partially met, for survival
2. Safety and security needs—things that make a person feel safe and comfortable
3. Love and belonging needs—the need to give and receive love and affection
4. Esteem needs—things that make people feel good about themselves; pride in abilities and accomplishments
5. Self-actualization needs—the need to continue to grow and change; working towards future goals.

The basic physical needs such as food, fluid, and oxygen are considered survival needs and must be met, or at least partially met, if life is to continue. They are the lowest level of needs and are usually partially satisfied before higher level needs. The nursing care of critically ill patients usually focuses on physiological needs. When the patient improves, when life is no longer threatened, the satisfaction of higher level needs gains in importance. Higher level needs begin with safety/security needs and continue through self-actualization needs.

Using Maslow's theory of basic needs, consider the following data and their relationship to a basic need:

1. **Physiological needs**
   —temperature 103°F.
   —respiration 36 per minute

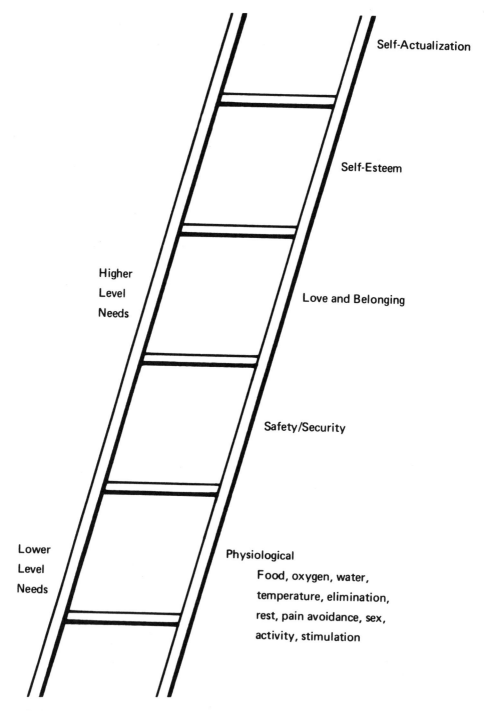

Self-Actualization

Self-Esteem

Higher
Level
Needs

Love and Belonging

Safety/Security

Lower
Level
Needs

Physiological
    Food, oxygen, water,
    temperature, elimination,
    rest, pain avoidance, sex,
    activity, stimulation

FIGURE 1–2.   Maslow's hierarchy of human needs.

  —liquid stool four times in one hour

  —complains of sharp continuous pain in right lower quadrant

 2. **Safety/security need**

  —sleeps with night light

  —"You won't forget me down in x-ray will you?"

  —"Last time I was in the hospital I got my

   roommate's pill by accident."

 3. **Love and belonging**

  —parents are with Billy (hospitalized child)

  —"We were married 40 years when my wife died. I miss her so

   much."

 4. **Self-esteem**

  —"I can't even control my bowels—just like a baby."

  —"I can't go to physical therapy without a shower and a shave."

 5. **Self-actualization**

  —"My children are grown with families of their own. Raising

   them has been my biggest accomplishment."

  —"Teaching nursing students is more than a job. I feel like I'm

   contributing to their development and to the profession."

  —"There is so much to learn about caring for my baby."

The data recorded within each category may indicate the current status of need satisfaction, alterations in meeting the need, or perhaps interferences in meeting the need. By collecting data in each of these need categories, the nurse develops a format for systematically considering the total patient rather than viewing an illness or a symptom. Comprehensive nursing care results from a consideration of the total patient. At the end of this chapter there is an assessment form that uses Maslow's hierarchy of needs as an organizing framework.

Henderson's Components of Nursing Care. Another framework which may be used to structure the nursing admission assessment was developed by nurse author Virginia Henderson. She described 14 needs or components of nursing care that a nurse may help the patient to perform:

 1. Breathe normally

 2. Eat and drink adequately

 3. Eliminate body waste

 4. Move and maintain desirable posture

 5. Sleep and rest

 6. Select suitable clothing, dress and undress

 7. Maintain body temperature

   8. Keep the body clean and well groomed and protect the integument
   9. Avoid dangers in the environment and avoid injuring others
   10. Communicate with others
   11. Worship according to one's faith
   12. Work in such a way that there is a sense of accomplishment
   13. Play, or participate in various forms of recreation
   14. Learn, discover, or satisfy the curiosity that leads to "normal" development and health, and use available health facilities (Henderson, 1978).

After reading Henderson's list of nursing activities, the nurse can readily adapt the list to a data collection format. For example, the following questions and observations relate to Henderson's activities:

Activity 1. Breathe normally. The nurse counts the respirations, observes the depth of breathing, presence of retractions or nasal flaring, and uses a stethoscope to listen for lung sounds. The nurse may also ask the patient such questions as: Do you ever feel short of breath? What activity causes this? Do you have any allergies that make you congested or that make it difficult to breathe? Do you ever experience nosebleeds? The nurse also examines the nailbeds and extremities for color, warmth, and capillary refill. All of these observations indicate the level of oxygenation.

Activity 2. Eat and drink normally. The nurse may ask the patient to describe a normal day's diet, when the major meal of the day is taken, foods that cause the patient problems, and to describe the resulting problems. The height, weight, and triceps skinfold may all be measured as a part of these data.

Gordon's Functional Health Patterns. A third schema that is being used to structure nursing assessment is functional health pattern typology developed by Gordon (1982) (see Appendix A-Care Plan #1). Gordon proposes that the nurse assess the response pattern of the patient in eleven areas and then evaluate to determine if the pattern is functional or dysfunctional for a particular patient. The functional patterns specified by Gordon include:

   1. Health-Perception Health Management Pattern
   2. Nutritional-Metabolic Pattern
   3. Elimination Pattern
   4. Activity-Exercise Pattern
   5. Sleep-Rest Pattern
   6. Cognitive-Perceptual Pattern

7. Self-Perception Self-Concept Pattern
8. Role-Relationship Pattern
9. Sexuality-Reproductive Pattern
10. Coping-Stress-Tolerance Pattern
11. Value-Belief Pattern.

NANDA'S Human Response Patterns. Another structure that may yield a future assessment format is the proposal by the North American Nursing Diagnosis Association (NANDA) (see Appendix A-Care Plan #2). This is an international group which has provided leadership in an effort to develop nursing diagnoses. The purpose of the organization is to develop, refine, and promote a taxonomy of nursing diagnoses terminology of general use to professional nurses (NANDA Bylaws: Article 1, Section 2) (Carroll-Johnson, 1989). Taxonomy here refers to an orderly classification of nursing diagnoses. NANDA proposes classifying nursing diagnoses using nine human response patterns (Taxonomy 1 Revised, June 1988): Exchanging, Communication, Relating, Valuing, Choosing, Moving, Perceiving, Knowing, and Feeling. Nursing diagnoses are then organized under each of these patterns. With further development, this approach may yield a powerful assessment tool for nursing.

Human Growth and Development. Any format used for data collection is acceptable as long as it is thorough, comprehensive, and considers both the physiological and psychosocial aspects of the human being. In addition, any data collection approach must also include consideration of the individual's level of growth and development. Each chronological age has corresponding developmental tasks, both physical and psychosocial. A developmental task may be thought of as a job, a hurdle, a challenge, or an accomplishment related to a particular chronological age span. Illness may interfere with completion of developmental tasks appropriate to an age span or with progression to the next developmental level. During illness an individual may even regress to an earlier level of development. For example, the 3-year-old who has been toilet trained for 6 months may begin bed wetting again during hospitalization. The adolescent who has been menstruating for 6 months may cease to menstruate during a lengthy confinement in a body cast. Other individuals may appear to arrest at a developmental level during the stress of illness and hospitalization. For example, an infant may fail to begin to crawl and stand during illness. The infant may remain at the developmental level achieved prior to hospitalization and show very little new learning until the stress of hospitalization and illness is reduced.

Thus it is important for nurses to include assessment of developmental levels and tasks associated with each stage so they can recognize and understand variations from normal age-related development in patients. By recognizing that a child is regressing to an earlier level or is failing to keep up with peers' development, the nurse may be able to work with parents and other hospital staff to reduce the damaging influence that hospitalization is having on that child's development. The nurse who has a knowledge of developmental levels and the associated tasks will be able to further individualize nursing care. For example, adolescent developmental tasks focus on self-identity. While caring for adolescents, the nurse might choose a nonauthoritative approach which would allow the patient the maximum amount of choice. Similarly, a school-age child's developmental level focuses on independence and project completion. Nursing care that encourages the child's self-care will promote developmental growth. Table 1-2 is a brief summary of some of the major developmental tasks corresponding to chronological age.

Table 1–2   Major Developmental Tasks

1. Infancy—1 month to 1 year
   —developing a sense of trust and belonging from relationship with mother and father
   —differentiating self from environment
   —learning to eat solid foods, to walk, to explore, to communicate
2. Toddler—1–3 years
   —developing will power, independence
   —learning to feed self, to run, communicate verbally, control elimination
   —exploring environment
3. Preschool—3–6 years
   —developing sexual identity
   —developing sense of initiative
   —working on autonomy, dressing self, washing
   —developing sense of time, space, distance
   —developing imagination
   —playing cooperatively
4. School age—6 to puberty
   —developing a sense of work; planning and carrying out projects
   —learning the skills for survival in the child's culture
   —developing modesty
   —learning to read, to calculate
   —developing neuromuscular coordination
   —learning to control emotions
5. Adolescent—12–20 years
   —developing physical maturity
   —developing autonomy from home and family

—developing self-identity
—coping with body image changes
—identifying with peer group
6. Young adulthood—18–40 years
—establishment of enduring close physical and emotional relationships
—child bearing, child rearing
—establishing financial security
—community responsibility
—social interaction with peers
7. Middle adult—40–65 years of age
—separation from children
—establishment in job
—adapt to aged parents
—adapt to physiological changes of aging
—adjustment to altered relationship with spouse
8. Older adult
—Acceptance of own life as valuable and appropriate
—Adaptation to reduced physical health and strength
—Possible death of spouse
—Adjustment to retirement income
—Development of relationships with new family members
—Adaptation to change in living location and style

Data Collection Skills

At the time the patient is admitted to the hospital, the nurse begins planning nursing care for the patient. This is begun using the skills of data collection. Observation, interview, and examination are three methods the nurse uses to collect data. Although there are multiple sources the nurse may use for data collection, the patient is always the primary source. Even if the patient is unable to communicate verbally, the nurse can elicit valuable data using observation and examination skills. Additional data sources may be the patient's past medical record (chart), family members, and other persons giving care to the patient. Professional journals, reference texts, and clinical nurse specialists are also important sources of data.

Nursing observations result in objective data. *Objective data* are factual data that are observed by the nurse and could be noted by any other skilled observer. During the assessment phase of the nursing process the nurse describes the signs or behaviors observed without drawing conclusions or making interpretations. At this point the nurse focuses on establishing a comprehensive data base about the patient. Premature interpretation and analysis based on incomplete data may lead to errors. See Table 1-3 for examples of objective data. The column of judgments and conclusions

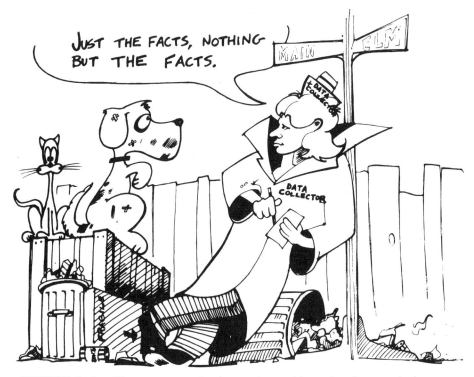

FIGURE 1–3.   The nurse records observations without drawing conclusions.

demonstrates the interpretations of one individual nurse. Consider that "neatly groomed" may mean different things to different individuals, whereas "hair combed, makeup applied" is concise and descriptive.

Contrasted with objective data are subjective data. *Subjective data* are information given verbally by the patient. Examples of this type of data are the following statements:

"I feel so nervous."

"My stomach is burning."

"I want to be alone now."

From the examples of subjective data listed above each nurse could infer many different interpretations. For example, the nurse might guess that the patient is nervous, fearing a diagnosis of cancer. This interpretation is not justified on the basis of the patient's statement. The patient could be nervous for many different reasons. The task during data collection is merely to observe, collect, and record data. Subjective data such as

Table 1–3   Objective Data

Objective Data	Judgments and Conclusions
Hair combed, makeup applied	Improved body image
Drags right leg when walking	Intoxicated
Tremors of both hands	Patient very afraid
250 cc dark amber urine	Voided large amount
Patient in bed, covers over head, facing wall; no verbal response to questions	Patient depressed
Administered own 8 A.M. insulin using sterile technique	Understands self-administration of insulin
Ate cereal, juice, toast, coffee	Good appetite
Requests pain med q2h	Low pain tolerance

the examples in Table 1-4 are best recorded as direct quotes, thus providing the reader with the original information.

Observation.   Observation is a high level nursing skill that requires a great deal of practice. Consider a grocery shopping trip. Even though it is possible to have shopped the store several times previously, few people can successfully recall all the items they need without a list or even find the location of all of the items they wish to purchase. The skills of observation and recall are difficult, but like all other skills they can be learned with systematic study and practice. The inexperienced student nurse will find it hard to perform nursing tasks and simultaneously continue the observation process. Yet it is this ability to perform constant, ongoing observations that is essential to assessment. For example, nursing students giving a first bedbath are concentrating so hard on the task that they may be

Table 1–4   Subjective Data

Subjective Data	Judgments and Conclusions
"Get out of my room."	Patient is hostile
"I know something is wrong with my baby."	Patient is anxious
"This catheter is killing me."	Patient has pain
"Where am I? How did I get here?"	Patient is confused
"I'm afraid they will find cancer when they operate."	Patient worried about surgery

---

Observation is a high level nursing skill . . .

"What you want are facts, not opinions—for who can have any opinion of any value as to whether the patient is better or worse, excepting the constant medical attendant, or the really observing nurse? The most important practical lesson that can be given to nurses is to teach them what to observe-how to observe-what symptoms indicate improvement-what the reverse, which are of importance-which are of non-which are the result of neglect-and what kind of neglect."   *p. 105*

"But if you can not get the habit of observation one way or the other, you had better give up the being a nurse, for it is not your calling, however kind and anxious you may be."   *p. 113*

"In dwelling upon the importance of sound observation, it must never be lost sight of what observation is for. It is not for the sake of piling up miscellaneous information or curious facts, but for the sake of saving life and increasing health and comfort."   *p. 125*

Florence Nightingale *Notes On Nursing: What It Is and What It Is Not.* From an unabridged republication of the first American edition as published in 1860. (1969) New York: Dover Publications.

---

unable to make observations or converse with the patient. As students gain skill in giving physical care, they can shift their attention to the total patient and begin to collect data through observation. They are now able to observe the skin condition, color, and temperature while bathing a patient. The quality, depth, and effort of respirations can be noted. The ability of the patient to move, as well as any pain associated with movement is noted. While giving a backrub, the skilled student can view the skin over the lower back, which is often an area of breakdown. The condition of the mucous membrane is noted during oral hygiene. The ability of the patient to tolerate activity may also be observed as the nurse watches for signs of fatigue during and after the bath.

Interview.   The interview is a structured form of communication that the nurse uses to collect data. Both the ability to ask questions and the ability to listen are essential to successful interviews.

The nursing history or nursing admission assessment is one type of interview. This is completed by the nurse at the time of admission. The focus of the nursing history is the patient's response to actual or potential health problems. As a part of this, the nurse reviews the patient's past health history and coping methods that have been effective or ineffective. Data related to the patient's life-style may also help to identify health risk factors. The nursing history is not a duplicate of the medical history, which has the disease process as its main focus. The purpose of the nursing history is to enable the nurse to plan nursing care for the patient. The nurse clearly and directly conveys this purpose to the patient at the beginning of the interview. The nurse may say something like, "Mr. Jones, I am Ms. Murray. I am the registered nurse who will be responsible for planning the nursing care you will receive while you are here. I would like to spend about a half hour with you now talking about your health history and completing this nursing admission form. This information will help me to work with you to begin to plan your nursing care." Note that the nurse has introduced herself in a professional manner and has clearly stated her professional accountability. If the institution uses them, this would be the appropriate time for the nurse to give the patient a business card which also indicates a hospital telephone number where messages may be left when the nurse is not on the unit. This introduction is in contrast to, "Hi, I'm Anne and I'm your nurse. I need to ask you some questions."

Prior to beginning the nursing history, the nurse helps to make the patient as comfortable as possible. This would include assessing for pain and doing what is necessary to reduce discomfort. It may also be helpful to offer the patient the opportunity to go to the bathroom before beginning. Note that the nurse in the above example also gave the patient some indication of the amount of time the interview would take. This is helpful to the patient who may be expecting visitors or perhaps planning to make a telephone call. The nurse may also offer the patient a beverage if medically permitted. This may help to put the patient at ease and contribute to openness in the interview process. It is also helpful if the nurse sits during the interview at a level where eye contact between the nurse and the patient can be easily maintained. This reduces the superior (nurse standing)-inferior (patient in bed) feeling of the nurse-patient relationship and conveys that the nurse has time to listen.

Most hospitals have a nursing history form that the nurse fills out on admission. This form guides or structures the interview, but the form is only a starting point. The nurse uses professional judgment to clarify areas of confusion or to elicit additional relevant data. The nurse does not form judgments or conclusions during the data collection phase, nor does the nurse rely on the judgments or conclusions of the patient. For example the nurse does not ask the patient, "Do you have problems with your bowel movements?'' To this question the patient may easily reply ''No.'' This illustrates a judgement made by the patient. Contrast this with the following dialogue between a nurse and a patient:

Nurse: What is your normal pattern of bowel movements (BM)?
Patient: I have a BM about every other day.
Nurse: Has this changed since you broke your hip?
Patient: Yes—I feel constipated almost all the time.
Nurse: Have you done anything to treat your constipation?
Patient: Yes—I started to take a laxative both in the morning and in the evening. Sometimes it works too much and I get diarrhea and other times I still feel constipated.

In this case the nurse has asked a series of open-ended questions (questions which may not be answered by yes or no) to assess the patient's health pattern and has elicited a more comprehensive picture of the health pattern. The beginning nurse may wish to use the following series of questions to guide the assessment of each health area (Table 1-5).

1. What is your normal pattern (or behavior)?
2. Has your current health problem (illness, injury) affected your normal pattern (or behavior)?
3. Have you done anything to help maintain or restore patterns (behavior) affected by your current health problem?

The nurse will probably find it helpful to take notes and actually complete most of the form during the interview process. Some explanation is always given to the patient. The nurse may say, ''Mr. Jones, I will be taking notes as we talk to make sure that I am accurate in recording this

Table 1–5 Open Ended Questions to Guide Assessment of Health Patterns

Focus	Nurse	Patient Example
1. Normal pattern	"What do you usually eat for breakfast?"	"I like eggs and toast with lots of butter."
2. Effect of medical problems	"Has this changed since you've had this problem?"	"Yes, I really get heartburn from this."
3. Coping strategies	"Have you done anything different to help this?"	"Well, mostly I just skip breakfast or eat plain cereal. That helps."

information.'' At the end of the interview it is helpful if the nurse summarizes the notes for the patient, especially those areas where the current health problem has affected function or behavior. This contributes to the sense of trust in the nurse-patient relationship and gives the patient the opportunity to add or correct data.

Frequently, beginning nursing students are uncomfortable eliciting a nursing history. Students often state that they feel they are prying into personal matters. Students may be reassured that the patient has the right to refuse to discuss any topic and that this right must be respected. When patients do choose to reveal personal data, nurses and students are responsible for assuring that the shared information remains confidential. Such data will remain within the context of the professional relationship and will be shared only with those who need the information to provide care.

The formal nursing interview is not primarily intended to be a treatment in and of itself, but is an organized format for data collection. Frequently, however, the patient has a need to express feelings or share things that are worrisome and the nursing interview provides the opportunity and the uninterrupted attention of the nurse.

The informal aspect of the nursing interview is the conversation between the nurse and the patient in the course of giving nursing care. The close relationship developed while the nurse is giving physical care frequently enables the patient to express concerns. The nurse who can skillfully give physical care is then free to simultaneously focus attention on what the patient is saying.

The planned, deliberate communication the nurse uses to help identify and meet the health care needs of the patient is called *therapeutic communication*. Like other nursing skills, therapeutic communication requires practice to be effective. It may be difficult for beginning nursing students to give physical care while simultaneously engaging in therapeutic communication. Often, for example, the nurse uses the time spent giving a bedbath as an opportunity for therapeutic communication. This is often an unhurried, private time for conversation between the nurse and the patient. With practice the nurse is able to focus on what the patient is saying. During this communication the nurse also continues to make observations.

At other times, the nurse will plan a period of time for the sole purpose of engaging in therapeutic communication. This, too, may be difficult for the beginning student who may feel uncomfortable approaching patients without a technical skill (such as taking a blood pressure) to ''do for'' the patient. Often therapeutic communication may be the most appropriate skill to offer the patient. This may be the case when a patient is afraid, discouraged, or has just been told of a serious diagnosis.

Often therapeutic communication may be the most appropriate skill to offer the patient . . .

I remember it as if it were yesterday—and it happened over 20 years ago! I was a third year student nurse in a diploma program and I was working 3–11:30 P.M. on a rehabilitation unit. Most patients on this unit had survived a major trauma and were transferred to the unit for rehabilitation. Most of the patients were paraplegic or quadraplegic with little hope of return of function.

On this particular evening I had completed most of my work settling patients for the night. One young man, John, was very restless. He had been injured in a manufacturing accident and was permanently paralyzed from the waist down. He was very handsome, intelligent, and recently married at age 26 years. I had given him a muscle relaxant, a back rub, and assisted with hygiene. Though he usually retired early and slept soundly, tonight he seemed troubled and moody, not his usual self. At 11:10 I walked past his room and noticing his light still on, I entered his room to find him staring at the ceiling. "How's it going, John?" I asked as I settled into a chair at his bedside. "Do you want some company?" He invited me to stay and admitted he was at "rock bottom." We talked a long time and in the conversation that followed he revealed that he and his wife had always wanted children, and that there was still the chance that physically he could father a child. "But," he confided, "what would a kid think of having a father in a wheelchair?"

I told him! For my father had multiple sclerosis and had suffered a progressively degenerative course to where he was ultimately a quadriplegic. I told him of the tough times, of the things I missed or envied in my friends' fathers, but I told him too of the love and support of my father . . . of the closeness of our relationship . . . of my respect for and pride in my father. "But," John said, "that was because you were a girl. What if I had a son?" I couldn't answer for my brother, I said, but I could describe my family life. After a long time, John said "Thank you, you've helped." I finished my charting and when I left the unit his light was out and he was sleeping.

Examination. The final activity of data collection is examination. A complete physical examination is a skill beyond the scope of most registered nurses and is usually a skill done by nurses with advanced education and training. A partial physical examination which is limited to an area of practice or which focuses on a specific problem is an expected skill of all nurses. Before beginning the physical process of examination, the nurse establishes a relationship with the patient. The nurse always precedes the examination with an explanation of the procedure and requests the patient's permission to proceed. The nurse always provides for the patient's privacy, closing doors and pulling curtains as necessary. The nurse checks with patients and asks if they would prefer if their visitors wait outside the room before beginning. The nurse might say something like, "Mrs. Jones, I'd like to do a physical examination now with your permission. If you feel any discomfort will you please tell me? I'll begin by checking your eyes and ears." When doing only a partial physical examination, the nurse might state, "I'd like to take a look at your stitches and the drain site to make sure everything is healing."

The nurse is then ready to begin a physical examination of the patient. The nurse may choose to conduct a total body assessment or to focus on one or more specific areas such as lung sounds, stitches, or a wound or a drain. If a patient complains of a generalized pain, the nurse may conduct a very thorough examination. In contrast, if a child in the emergency room fell from a bicycle and shows the nurse a large bleeding laceration on the elbow, this might be the initial focus of the examination. It is important that the nurse conducts a thorough examination as soon as possible since internal injuries which are not so readily apparent may also be present.

In obtaining this examination data, the nurse uses a systematic approach to avoid omissions. For nursing students, the particular curriculum of a school may require a certain approach. Hospitals may, by the forms they provide, structure the examination done by a practicing nurse. It really does not matter which approach is used as long as it is methodical and the nurse uses it consistently to gain a high degree of skill. One nurse may follow a cephalocaudal (head to toe) approach which begins with an assessment of the hair, skull, eyes, ears, nose, mouth, and facial skin and moves in a downward direction. Another nurse may select a body system approach which may begin with a consideration of the respiratory system, moving to the digestive system, to the cardiovascular system and so forth. Any methodical, thorough approach is acceptable as long as it meets the need to gather relevant data that helps to identify health problems requiring nursing intervention.

During physical examination, the nurse uses senses and skills to gather information about the patient. *Visualization* is inspection of the patient's body. This is coupled with the use of the senses such as hearing, smelling (certain disease processes or physical changes are associated with characteristic odors), and touching. Visualization is often the most appropriate starting place for a physical examination because the nurse will not cause the patient any discomfort. The nurse also uses the skill of *auscultation*, which includes listening with a stethoscope to heart, lung, and bowel sounds.

Next the nurse may palpate or feel the body. This may give the nurse information about organ position, body temperature, abnormal growths, abdominal rigidity, or the location of pain. Some nurses may be skilled in the use of *percussion,* the tapping of a body surface with a rubber-tipped mallet or with the fingers. This is done to elicit responses, usually in the form of sound or movement, that give information about an underlying body part. For example, it is common practice to percuss a distended abdomen for a drumlike sound indicating retained flatus (gas) in the bowel following abdominal surgical procedure.

While it is necessary to establish a relationship with the patient prior to examination, the examination itself can be a tool for showing concern and enhancing the relationship. The nurse who stops to palpate the abdomen and listen to bowel sounds when the patient complains of pain, shows concern for the patient, identifies possible changes in patient status, and establishes credibility. The observations the nurse makes during the examination are recorded as objective data: 3-inch scar, left lower quadrant; temperature 98.6°F; blood pressure (BP) 110/70; no bowel sounds present.

During the assessment phase the nurse has the potential to collect volumes of data about a patient. Throughout the process it is important to consider the significance of the data to the task at hand, which is identifying problems and planning nursing intervention. As the student practices data collection, skill is gained in eliciting and recording relevant data. It is also essential that the student learns to report data in a timely manner to the appropriate person. If the physician sees the patient once a day, and a major change in the patient's condition is noted after that visit, it is the responsibility of the nurse to report this immediately in addition to completing the necessary documentation.

SUMMARY

Assessment is the first step in the nursing process and the one step which is a part of every other step in the nursing process. The nursing assessment which the nurse completes upon the patient's admission to the hospital is focused on the patient's response to actual or potential health problems. During assessment the nurse collects data by interview, observation, and examination. The nurse does not make judgments or conclusions at this time but focuses on establishing a comprehensive data base which reflects the health status of the patient. Similarly the nurse seeks to gather only data, not judgments and conclusions, from the patient by the use of open questions: "What is your normal pattern of . . . ? Has it changed with illness? Are you doing anything to cope with the changes?"

PRACTICE EXERCISE

I.   Consider the following pieces of data and label them:
     O = objective
     S = subjective
     J = judgment or conclusions.

   1. 75 cc dark amber urine
   2. Patient is afraid of surgery because her mother died in the hospital.
   3. "I can't go that long (8 hours) without smoking."
   4. Large amount bright red drainage from incision site.
   5. Patient states that the pain is 8 on 1–10 scale.
   6. Respiratory rate of 36 after walking length of hall unassisted.
   7. Patient's oral intake is in excess of body requirements.
   8. Intelligent and articulate middle aged adult.
   9. Confused elderly white male.
   10. Patient is becoming increasingly agitated.

II. Given the following patient responses, formulate two additional questions the nurse might ask which would encourage the patient to provide more complete information about his or her response to actual or potential health problems.

   1. Patient is 86-year-old woman with arthritis, living alone in own home. You are to assess her mobility status.
      Nurse: "Do you have any problems getting around?"
      Patient: "Nope."
   2. Patient is 12-year-old boy with possible appendicitis. You are to assess pain.
      Nurse: "Are you having any pain?"
      Patient: "No—can I go home now?"
   3. Patient is 45-year-old woman, slightly overweight. You are to assess the patient's nutritional status.
      Nurse: "Do you have any nutritional problems?"
      Patient: "None other than eating too much."
   4. Patient is 53-year-old man admitted for possible heart attack. You are to assess the patient's coping skills/stress management.

Nurse: "Do you feel that you are under a lot of stress?"
Patient: "No more than most people."

5. Patient is 17-year-old high school football team captain admitted for diagnostic tests possibly for mononucleosis. You are initiating the nursing assessment.
Nurse: "How have you been feeling?"
Patient: "Not too bad."

ANSWERS TO EXERCISE ON ASSESSMENT

I.

1. O
2. J
3. S
4. J (Use of word large makes it a judgment.)
5. S

6. O
7. J
8. J
9. J
10. J (Describe the behaviors that made you label the patient agitated.)

II.

1. "Can you tell me how you manage things—like cooking and grocery shopping?"
"Has your arthritis made this hard for you to do?"
"What things have you figured out that help you?"

2. "It sounds like you want to get out of here. Have you ever been in a hospital before?"
"What was that like for you?"
"What did the nurses do then that helped you?"
"Do you think that if your side stops hurting you can go home?"

3. "Do you think you are eating too much?"
"Is this more difficult since you've been sick?"
"What has helped you in the past?"

4. "How much stress is normal for 'most people'?"
"How do you cope with stress?"
"Does it work for you?"

5. "What is 'not too bad' for you?"
"And what do you do when you feel like that?"
"Does that help?"
"What problems brought you into the hospital or to the doctor?"

CASE STUDY: DATA COLLECTION

The case study method will be used throughout this book to illustrate the steps of the nursing process. The same case study of Mrs. Witten will be found in each chapter to illustrate the various steps in the nursing process. The following pages illustrate the nursing assessment that was done for Mrs. Witten upon admission.

89714530
Witten, Laura
6/3/90 room 511
Dr. Ronal/Keller

NURSING ASSESSMENT

(Data Collection Format based on Maslow's Basic Needs framework)

General Information

Information given by: patient

Name: Mrs. Laura Witten

Age: 45 yrs   Sex: female   Race: Caucasian

Admission date/time: 6/3/90; 9 A.M.

Admitting medical diagnosis: Possible Cholecystitis/Cholelithiasis

Arrived on unit by: wheelchair   from: home

Accompanied by: husband

Admitting Weight/VS: T. 99.0, P. 96, R. 28, BP 138/88 ; 148 lbs, 5'4"

Patient's Perception of Reason for Admission: severe pain in right upper quadrant; "It has never been this bad before. I couldn't stand it at home. The doctor thinks it might be my gallbladder"

How has problem been managed by patient at home? "I took 2 aspirins but that just didn't help at all; it made me nauseated"

Allergies: no known allergies

Medications: ASA 10 gr for pain in abdomen; no prescription meds

Physiological Needs

Oxygenation: some restlessness, R. 28, reports no difficulty breathing; states nonsmoker; clear breath sounds; no cough; P. 96, strong and regular; no murmurs heard, denies any chest pain; brisk capillary refill of fingernail beds; no ankle or leg edema; skin pink but pale

Temperature Maintenance: T. 99.0; denies a fever in the last few days; states she feels warm

Nutritional–Fluid: 5'4", 148 lbs; states she has gained about 20 lbs over the last 5 years; states she has been eating regular meals (3 meals a day and occasional nighttime snack) and not dieting; reports food sometimes helps the discomfort; reports greasy or rich, buttery foods make her sick (nausea & vomiting); good skin turgor; has not eaten for 10 hours but has taken fluids; last intake one hour ago—large glass of gingerale and ice that she sipped and kept down; slight nausea now

Elimination: last bowel movement 6/3; normal pattern qod; denies stool hard or difficult to pass; denies any problem with urination; states normal large amounts every few hours, no burning

Rest–Sleep: usually retires at 10:30 P.M. and sleeps until 7 A.M.; states no problem sleeping at home but has never been in hospital and "with this pain I was not able to sleep much last night;" denies use of sleeping pills

Pain Avoidance: rates pain as an "8" on a 1–10 scale; says it started last night and has gotten worse; it is a continuous sharp pain in right upper quadrant; reports a few previous attacks over the last year which have lasted a few hours and then subsided; clenching hands and gritting teeth; restless

Sexuality–Reproductive: last menstrual period 5/20; states she is fairly regular on a 28–30 day cycle; denies use of any birth control, states husband had a vasectomy after the birth of their third child 7 years ago; denies any concerns with sexual aspect of her life or role as a woman

Stimulation–Activity: states she is active and has no problems; states she walks around the block occasionally; works part-time as a clerk in a children's store; enjoys TV

Safety–Security Needs

She is oriented and alert; responds appropriately to questions; states she wears glasses and really needs them; states she is "scared of being in the hospital and of being sick" and has never been in the hospital other than for the birth of her children; tears in eyes; diaphoretic, hands trembling; last PAP test was 2 years ago and negative; last breast exam 2 years ago, states she was never really taught breast self-exam and does not do it; husband here and plans to stay with her

Love–Belonging Needs
has 3 children; husband with her

Self-Esteem Needs
"I'm never sick; the doctor thinks it might be my gallbladder causing all the trouble. I don't mean to act like a baby but this pain is so bad; I was supposed to work today and the kids will be worried about me when they get home from school but Bob (husband) will be there today for them. They really count on me being there when they get home. 'MOM' is the first thing they holler when they come through the door after school"

Self-Actualization Needs
(No data.)

CHAPTER 2

Diagnosis

II. Nursing diagnoses are derived from the health status data. (Standards of Nursing Practice, American Nurses' Association, 1973)

Diagnosis is the second step in the nursing process and is the phase during which the nurse analyzes the data gathered during assessment and identifies problem areas for the patient. The nurse then makes a nursing diagnosis. The terms *nursing diagnosis* and *diagnosis* do not mean the same thing in this chapter and may be confusing for the student. *Diagnosis* is a process of data analysis and problem identification. It is a form of decision making which the nurse uses to arrive at judgments and conclusions about patients' responses to actual or potential health problems. A *nursing diagnosis* is the specific result of diagnosing and is the problem statement nurses use to communicate professionally. It refers to a problem statement that the nurse makes regarding a patient's condition. It is helpful to think of the term as a noun (nursing diagnosis) or verb (diagnose) to distinguish between the two.

There are three activities in the diagnosis step:

$$\text{Diagnosis} = \frac{\text{Data}}{\text{Analysis}} + \frac{\text{Problem}}{\text{Identification}} + \frac{\text{Formulation of}}{\text{Nursing Diagnosis}}$$

DATA ANALYSIS

Question: "So now that I've got all this data what do I do with it?"
Answer: "Make sense out of it and use it."

The nurse has completed the initial systematic data collection and is now ready to begin the process of analysis. The nurse begins the activity of data analysis by considering all the data that were gathered during the assessment phase of the nursing process. The nurse quickly checks for completeness of the data. For example, if the data were collected in a format which used Maslow's hierarchy of basic needs, it may be that data about rest and sleep patterns were unclear, incomplete, or omitted. The nurse may decide to go back and gather additional data as needed.

The nurse also looks for inconsistencies or ambiguity in the data. It may become apparent to the nurse that the sequence of events in the history is contradictory and needs to be resolved. Two data sources may also be inconsistent. For example, the patient may report having only an occasional "social drink" while the spouse gives data about "drinking 10–12 cans of beer daily." At this point no judgment is made about the existence of a problem but the inconsistency is noted. Another example might be that the nurse does not understand from reading the assessment what methods the patient has used for pain relief and with what result.

The data are evaluated for comprehensiveness—does the data give a complete picture of the patient considering both physical and psychosocial aspects of the person? The nurse asks whether the assessment has considered all areas that may be relevant to the patient. This considers such things as higher level needs, cultural factors, data related to growth and development, in addition to the more obvious physical areas. These factors taken all together comprise holistic health, that is, the concept that the mind and the body are inseparable and one cannot be treated without the other. In summary, the nurse reviews the data for clarity, consistency, completeness, and comprehensiveness.

After reviewing the data the nurse is ready to begin analysis. This is the process of studying the data and making judgments and conclusions about the meaning of the data. The nurse will decide if the data indicate a problem for the patient or a situation which puts the patient at risk for the development of problems in the future. The following decisions are made based on the data:

1. Determine whether measurement data are within the normal range for the patient and within the norms for that patient's age group. For example, if the nurse has taken the blood pressure of the patient, the nurse can now ask if this pressure is typical for this individual. The nurse also determines if this BP reading is within the normal range for this patient's age.

2. Determine if functioning described by the patient is typical of past functioning and within normal patterns for the patient's age. The nurse could consider the bowel elimination pattern which the patient reported as "every other day, soft and easy to pass, no blood, no use of laxatives but daily bran flakes, no change with diabetes" and decide that the pattern is both typical for the patient and within normal patterns for adults.

3.   Determine what relationships exist between pieces of data. For example, if the data reveal that the patient is 25% overweight, has an elevated blood pressure, and has no understanding of caloric content of food and body requirements, the nurse recognizes the relationship between the many factors affecting the obesity. Another patient may be unable to sleep, appear very anxious, be very demanding of the nurses' time, and have a history which includes a parent who died during a routine surgical procedure. While the obvious interpretation that the patient is also worried about dying during surgery needs confirmation by the patient, it seems clear that there is a relationship between the data.

4.   Evaluate the physical assessment data as positive, negative, normal, or abnormal signs or findings. For example, if the nurse has completed auscultation of the patient's lungs, the nurse makes a decision if the findings were normal or not and if not, which abnormality was heard and the location of the abnormal sound. This is clearly recorded. Similarly the decision that a particular aspect of the examination was negative is valuable because it notes that a judgment has been made and a problem ruled out. These decisions may be difficult for the beginning nurse to make. Until the nurse has had a lot of experience, it is difficult to judge what are normal versus what are abnormal lung sounds. The student should not hesitate to ask a more experienced nurse to assist in this evaluation.

5.   Determine whether specific behavior patterns contribute to the health and well-being of the client. The nurse may evaluate that dietary and exercise patterns of the client foster cardiovascular health as in the case of the patient who reports that she has never smoked, has decreased her intake of red meat to twice a week, and walks two miles a day several times a week. The nurse considers the opposite decision in the case of the patient who reports that she is a pack a day smoker, "my father died of a heart attack," needs to lose 30 pounds, and has no physical activity. Here the nurse would also try to determine if the patient perceives these things to be problematic and if the patient is willing to make any life-style changes. While the nurse may evaluate something to be a problem, the adult patient always has the right to make a decision to refuse the health professional's recommendations. Although this may generate feelings of ineffectiveness and frustration in the nurse, it is the goal of health education to assist the patient in making informed decisions and it is the patient's right to make the decisions.

6.   Determine the strengths and resources, as well as limitations, the

patient possesses which affect health status. This may include such things as cognitive abilities or potential, willingness to change, family support, economic resources, and available time to invest. For example, a nursing student who is going to school full-time and working part-time would probably have little time, energy, or money to invest in an exercise club. For another patient, the nurse may make the judgment that the YMCA membership the patient holds is a valuable resource affecting health status. Another patient who has suffered a mild heart attack may state, "That was a warning. Now I am ready to do whatever I have to, to get healthy and stay healthy." The nurse may interpret that as a willingness to receive health teaching and a motivation to follow through.

PROBLEM IDENTIFICATION

The next step is to identify a broad focus area requiring nursing intervention, such as nutrition, elimination, or incorrect or inadequate information. This is the identification of a problem area. Nurses use both nursing theory, general knowledge base, and cumulative experience to define this area. For example, in a patient who is a newly diagnosed non-insulin dependent diabetic the nurse may read data that includes such things as: a history of being overweight since childhood, "My Mother used to bake me a chocolate whipped cream cake if I got a good report card," "I've tried every diet in the book," "I don't feel jolly—aren't fat people supposed to be jolly?," "My children are plump but it is just baby fat and they'll grow out of it," patient is 43 years old, 5'2", weight 189 lbs. The nurse uses a knowledge of human growth and development, behavioral psychology, anatomy and physiology, and nursing in considering these data. A focus for nursing intervention in the area of nutrition is indicated.

In a second example, another patient may include the following data: pain in the lower back, unable to perform job (cashier in grocery store) because it causes pain, unable to do any housework without aggravation of pain, "I'm no use to anybody," "My Mother had a bad back and she was an invalid at age 45." Here the nurse also uses the knowledge of sciences related to nursing to recognize that the data indicate an area for nursing intervention. The nurse identifies the back pain as the most immediate problem focus area requiring intervention although there is data to indicate that the patient is also experiencing low self-esteem.

After a broad focus area is chosen, a narrower, more specific problem statement is selected from the diagnostic statements developed by NANDA.

NURSING DIAGNOSIS:

is a statement of a present or potential patient problem that requires nursing intervention in order to be resolved, lessened, or adapted to.

At this point the student may choose to consult the *Nursing Diagnosis Pocketbook* which is included with this text. Table 2-1 lists the problem focus areas corresponding approximately to basic human needs. Specific problem statements developed by NANDA are listed under each focus area. Alternatively the student may use Table 2-2 which is an alphabetized listing of NANDA diagnostic categories. These are organized according to nine human response patterns as a broad focus area.

Table 2–1   Nursing Diagnoses Organized by Basic Human Need

1. **Oxygen Needs**
   — Altered (specify) tissue perfusion (renal, cerebral, cardiopulmonary, gastrointestinal, peripheral)
   —Decreased cardiac output
   —Impaired gas exchange
   —Ineffective airway clearance
   —Ineffective breathing pattern
   —Potential for aspiration
   —Potential for suffocation
2. **Temperature Maintenance**
   —Potential altered body temperature
   —Hypothermia
   —Hyperthermia
   —Ineffective thermoregulation
3. **Nutritional and Fluid Needs**
   —Altered nutrition: Less than body requirements
   —Altered nutrition: More than body requirements
   —Altered nutrition: Potential for more than body requirements
   —Fluid volume deficit (1) (Regulatory failure)
   —Fluid volume deficit (2) (Active loss)
   —Potential fluid volume deficit
   —Fluid volume excess
   —Feeding self-care deficit
   —Impaired swallowing
   —Ineffective breast-feeding
4. **Elimination Needs**
   —Constipation
   —Perceived constipation

—Colonic constipation
—Diarrhea
—Bowel incontinence
—Altered patterns of urinary elimination
—Stress incontinence
—Reflex incontinence
—Urge incontinence
—Functional incontinence
—Total incontinence
—Urinary retention
—Toileting self-care deficit

5. **Rest and Sleep Needs**
   —Fatigue
   —Sleep pattern disturbance
6. **The Need for Pain Avoidance**
   —Pain
   —Chronic pain
7. **Sexual Needs**
   —Sexual dysfunction
   —Altered sexuality patterns
8. **Stimulation Needs**
   —Activity intolerance
   —Potential activity intolerance
   —Diversional activity deficit
   —Impaired physical mobility
   —Unilateral neglect
   —Potential for disuse syndrome
   —Sensory/perceptual alterations (specify: visual, auditory, kinesthetic, gustatory, tactile, olfactory)
9. **Safety and Security Needs**
   Physiological level
   —Potential for infection
   —Dysreflexia
   —Potential for injury
   —Potential for poisoning
   —Potential for trauma
   —Impaired tissue integrity
   —Altered oral mucous membrane
   —Impaired skin integrity
   —Potential impaired skin integrity
   —Impaired home maintenance management
   —Altered health maintenance
   Higher level
   —Anxiety
   —Decisional conflict (specify)
   —Fear
   —Knowledge deficit

Table 2–1   Nursing Diagnoses Organized by Basic Human Need
(*Cont.*)

—Noncompliance
—Ineffective individual coping
—Ineffective denial
—Ineffective family coping: Disabling
—Ineffective family coping: Compromised
—Altered thought process
—Potential for violence: Self-directed or directed at others
—Post trauma response
—Rape-trauma syndrome
—Rape-trauma syndrome: Compound reaction
—Rape-trauma syndrome: Silent reaction

10. Love and Belonging Needs
—Impaired social interaction
—Social isolation
—Impaired verbal communication
—Altered parenting
—Potential altered parenting
—Altered family processes
—Parental role conflict
—Anticipatory grieving
—Dysfunctional grieving

11. Spiritual Needs
—Spiritual distress (distress of the human spirit)

12. Self-Esteem Needs
—Body image disturbance
—Bathing/hygiene self-care deficit
—Dressing/grooming self-care deficit
—Self-esteem disturbance
—Chronic low self-esteem
—Situational low self-esteem
—Altered role performance
—Personal identity disturbance
—Hopelessness
—Powerlessness
—Defensive coping

13. Self-Actualization Needs
—Family coping: Potential for growth
—Health seeking behavior
—Impaired adjustment
—Altered growth and development

Adapted from: *Classification of the Eighth Conference,* Proceedings of the Eighth Conference, edited by Rose Mary Carroll-Johnson. Philadelphia, Lippincott, 1989.

Table 2–2   Approved NANDA Nursing Diagnostic Categories. Listed by Human Response Pattern.

Pattern 1: Exchanging
   Altered nutrition: More than body requirements
   Altered nutrition: Less than body requirements
   Altered nutrition: Potential for more than body requirements
   Potential for infection
   Potential altered body temperature
   Hypothermia
   Hyperthermia
   Ineffective thermoregulation
   Dysreflexia
   Constipation
   Perceived constipation
   Colonic constipation
   Diarrhea
   Bowel incontinence
   Altered patterns of urinary elimination
   Stress incontinence
   Reflex incontinence
   Urge incontinence
   Functional incontinence
   Urinary retention
   Altered (specify) tissue perfusion (renal, cerebral, cardiopulmonary gastrointes-
      tinal, peripheral)
   Fluid volume excess
   Fluid volume deficit (1)
   Fluid volume deficit (2)
   Potential fluid volume deficit
   Decreased cardiac output
   Impaired gas exchange
   Ineffective airway clearance
   Ineffective breathing pattern
   Potential for injury
   Potential for suffocation
   Potential for poisoning
   Potential for trauma
   Potential for aspiration
   Potential for disuse syndrome
   Impaired tissue integrity
   Altered oral mucous membrane
   Impaired skin integrity
   Potential impaired skin integrity
Pattern 2: Communicating
   Impaired verbal communication

Table 2–2   Approved NANDA Nursing Diagnostic Categories. Listed by Human Response Pattern (*Cont.*)

Pattern 3: Relating
   Impaired social interaction
   Social isolation
   Altered role performance
   Altered parenting
   Potential altered parenting
   Sexual dysfunction
   Altered family process
   Parental role conflict
   Altered sexuality patterns
Pattern 4: Valuing
   Spiritual distress (distress of the human spirit)
Pattern 5: Choosing
   Ineffective individual coping
   Impaired adjustment
   Defensive coping
   Ineffective denial
   Ineffective family coping: Disabling
   Ineffective family coping: Compromised
   Family coping: Potential for growth
   Noncompliance (specify)
   Decisional conflict (specify)
   Health seeking behaviors (specify)
Pattern 6: Moving
   Impaired physical mobility
   Activity intolerance
   Fatigue
   Potential activity intolerance
   Sleep pattern disturbance
   Diversional activity deficit
   Impaired home maintenance management
   Altered health maintenance
   Feeding self-care deficit
   Impaired swallowing
   Ineffective breast-feeding
   Bathing/hygiene self-care deficit
   Dressing/grooming self-care deficit
   Toileting self-care deficit
   Altered growth and development
Pattern 7: Perceiving
   Body image disturbance
   Self-esteem disturbance
   Chronic low self-esteem
   Situational low self-esteem
   Personal identity disturbance

Sensory/perceptual alterations (specify: visual, auditory, kinesthetic, gustatory,
   tactile, olfactory)
Unilateral neglect
Hopelessness
Powerlessness
Pattern 8: Knowing
Knowledge deficit (specify)
Altered thought process
Pattern 9: Feeling
Pain
Chronic pain
Dysfunctional grieving
Anticipatory grieving
Potential for violence: Self-directed or directed at others
Post trauma response
Rape-trauma syndrome
Rape-trauma syndrome: Compound reaction
Rape-trauma syndrome: Silent reaction
Anxiety
Fear

From: *Classification of Nursing Diagnoses: Proceedings of the Eighth Conference,* edited
by Rose Mary Carroll-Johnson. Philadelphia, Lippincott, 1989.

FORMULATING THE NURSING DIAGNOSIS

The final activity in the process of diagnosis is the formulation of the
nursing diagnosis.

The definition above assumes that the problems the nurse chooses to
address are within the scope of the legal practice of nursing since this
assumption underlies all professional activity. The privileges granted by
licensure vary from state to state, country to country. Nurses with advanced degrees may be licensed to perform additional nursing care. However, all professional nurses share the responsibility of making nursing
diagnoses within their practice.

A nursing diagnosis is not the same as a medical diagnosis though it
may involve the medical diagnosis or treatment as a cause. For example,
the nursing diagnosis of *pain* is clearly caused by the medical diagnosis in
many cases: pain may be caused by a surgical incision, by cancer which
has metastasized to the bones, by stones in the gallbladder. However, since
nurses cannot treat the medical diagnosis, the direction for nursing diagnosis must then come from the problem part of the statement. Table 2-3
compares medical and nursing diagnoses. A medical diagnosis frequently

Table 2–3

A Nursing Diagnosis	
Is	*Is Not*
A statement of a patient problem	A medical diagnosis
Actual, potential, or possible	A nursing action
Within the scope of nursing practice	A physician order
Directive of nursing intervention	A therapeutic treatment

suggests nursing diagnoses. The experienced nurse who has cared for several patients with the same medical diagnosis will be able to predict some frequently occurring nursing diagnoses for a given medical condition. The nurse is then looking for data to confirm or disconfirm the prediction. This experience contributes to skill in making nursing diagnoses. Table 2-4 gives examples of nursing diagnoses which are suggested by medical diagnoses.

The nurse begins the process of writing nursing diagnoses by reviewing the problem focus area identified in the previous step. Does the focus area represent a problem? By definition, a diagnosis must be a problem for the patient. If it is not a problem, no diagnosis need be made. Consider the bowel function status of a patient restricted to bed rest. If the patient has a soft, formed stool without exertion every two or three days, elimination is not a problem and no nursing diagnosis need be made. However, the nurse also considers who defines the problem. If the patient considers it abnormal not to have a bowel movement daily and continues to express anxiety related to this, a problem does exist as defined by the patient. The nurse understands that physiologically no problem exists, but that the pa-

Table 2–4   Medical Diagnoses which Suggest Nursing Diagnoses

Medical Diagnosis	*Nursing Diagnosis*
Myocardial infarction	Fear related to possible recurrence and uncertain outcome
Chronic ulcerative colitis	Diarrhea related to CUC as manifested by 10–12 loose, watery, foul smelling stools per day
Chronic ulcerative colitis	Alteration in nutrition: less than body requirements related to altered G.I. absorption secondary to CUC.
Cancer of the breast	Potential body image disturbance if mastectomy is required
Cerebral vascular accident	Self-care deficit: dressing and grooming related to right sided flaccidity

tient could benefit from teaching regarding normal body function. Nursing care may then focus on teaching as an intervention tool to reduce anxiety. Nursing diagnoses may also identify growth areas for the patient. Many nurses in industrial health or occupational health nursing report that the clients they see are requesting ways to improve their health status. While this does not constitute a problem, it is a focus area for nursing intervention. Tripp and Stachowiak (1989) have proposed a nursing diagnosis that would label this as "health seeking behavior." This nursing diagnosis does clearly identify an area of nursing intervention that is not a problem in the negative sense.

Types of Nursing Diagnoses

Actual Nursing Diagnoses. As defined here, the problem expressed in the nursing diagnosis may be either actual or potential. An *actual nursing diagnosis* refers to a situation existing in the here and now. A patient on a general diet with a good appetite who has not had a bowel movement for four days, complains of low abdominal pain, and is unable to pass stool. This patient is constipated and requires assistance. This situation requires that an actual nursing diagnosis be made.

Potential Nursing Diagnoses. A *potential nursing diagnosis* refers to a problem which may develop in the future. The nurse has identified factors in either the admission data base or in ongoing assessments that indicate risk factors for the development of a problem. By identifying a potential problem, the nurse may be able to prevent the problem or to lessen its consequences. If a patient is on absolute bed rest while in a full leg cast, the patient is at risk for skin breakdown (decubitus ulcers) caused by inactivity, decreased circulation, and rubbing from the cast. Understanding the physiological effect of bedrest, the nurse may take action to prevent skin breakdown. In this case the problem is a potential one that requires preventive nursing action. The potential nursing diagnosis is made based on the nurse's learning and past experience in similar situations and on an understanding of pathophysiology. The problem would predictably occur without nursing intervention.

Possible Nursing Diagnoses. In still other situations the nurse may decide to formulate a tentative or *possible nursing diagnosis*. This may be compared to the physician who lists several "rule out" medical diagnoses in a patient's admission assessment. The physician may then order diagnostic tests to gather more data to make a decision. So it is with a possible nursing diagnosis. By considering a possible nursing diagnosis, the nurse assures continued collection of relevant data. With an increased data base, the nurse may be able to firmly establish the possible nursing diagnosis as valid or to eliminate it as invalid for a particular patient. For example:

> An adolescent has arrived in the emergency room to receive stitches for a scalp laceration. Treatment requires that a large portion of her head be shaved. The nurse considers a possible nursing diagnosis of situational low self-esteem related to loss of hair. The nurse bases this possible nursing diagnosis on a knowledge of growth and development, since most adolescents are very concerned about their physical appearance. Note, however, that this nursing diagnosis is not yet supported by data from the patient. The diagnosis at this point is based on inference and thus is only "possible." The nurse seeks to gather more data as she asks the patient, "A lot of girls would be very upset about having their hair cut. How do you feel about this?" The patient replies, "No problem. I can wear a wig a lot. Now if it had been a scar on my face—that I would have trouble with." The nurse then eliminated the possible nursing diagnosis.

COLLABORATIVE PROBLEMS

Some nurses also distinguish between nursing diagnoses which the nurse treats independently and those which the nurse treats collaboratively (jointly shared) with the physician. Nursing and medicine are complementary to each other. Physicians rely on nurses to understand and assess for physiological complications related to patients' medical treatments such as postsurgical phlebitis. The nurse and the physician discuss the problem and the physician will order new treatments, medications, or intensive monitoring. The nurse carries out these medical orders and continues assessment which is reported to the physician. These types of problems are collaborative. The nurse in this situation is not licensed to prescribe the primary treatment needed to resolve the problem. Much of the assessment and treatment of the problem is directed by the physician even though the nurse may carry it out and adapt it to the particular client situation. A large part of nursing care involves this kind of collaborative assessment and intervention. In contrast the independent role of the nurse deals with how the patient responds to actual or potential health problems. The nurse not only monitors the patient for these problems but is licensed to diagnose, prescribe, and carry out treatment for these problems. This text focuses on nursing diagnoses which are the independent responsibility of the nurse and are within the practice realm of professional nursing.

Many nursing diagnoses have both an independent aspect and a collaborative component. For example, there are many measures the nurse may independently use to assist the patient in pain (massage, guided imagery, relaxation techniques) although it is usually a physician prerogative to order a medication. (Some states permit nurse practitioners this practice privilege.) This is an example of a collaborative problem which incorporates independent nursing functions. Other collaborative problems are primarily within the realm of medicine and the nurse monitors the patient and reports to the physician for medical diagnoses and treatment. Fluid volume deficit is being discussed as such a collaborative problem. Even though this is a NANDA approved nursing diagnosis, much of the treatment is determined by the physician and implemented by the nurse. The physician orders the IV and electrolyte replacement, diet therapy, and activity levels but the nurse is responsible for the implementation. Much of the work of staff nurses in hospitals involves a collaborative role not only with physicians but with professionals in many other disciplines. Nurses share a collaborative role with therapeutic dieticians to resolve the nutritional problems of patients. Psychiatric nurses identify collaborative problems with dance therapists, music therapists, and occupational therapists. The collaborative role is not unique to the disciplines of nursing and medicine.

In addition to deciding if the focus area represents a problem for the patient, now the nurse considers a second criterion: does the problem require nursing intervention to be resolved, lessened, or accommodated to? The nurse may identify problems that are clearly within the realm of another health professional. In such case the nurse communicates the data to that professional and does not make a diagnosis.

Writing Nursing Diagnoses

Actual Nursing Diagnoses.   The following formula will result in a clear, concise statement of an *actual (or present) nursing diagnosis:*

> **Actual Nursing Diagnosis** = Patient Problem + Cause if Known

When writing the diagnosis the plus symbol is usually replaced by the words "related to" which are abbreviated "r/t". The following are examples of nursing diagnoses in this format:

Actual nursing diagnoses		
Problem	+	*Cause*
1. Impaired skin integrity	r/t	immobility
2. Parental role conflict	r/t	divorce
3. Impaired verbal communication	r/t	cultural differences

This is a very clear and concise way of writing nursing diagnoses. This is the way nursing diagnoses will usually be written in the hospital. The nurse may not always know the cause of the problem and in such a case may simply write "cause unknown."

PES Format.   There is another format used for writing actual nursing diagnoses which may be especially helpful for beginning nursing students. Using this approach, which is referred to as PES (Gordon, 1982), the formula for a nursing diagnosis would look like this:

PES APPROACH

P   +   E   +   S
Nursing Diagnosis = Problem + Etiology + Signs & Symptoms

Using this formula the nurse first selects the approved NANDA nursing diagnosis and then relates it to the cause which is the same as the etiology. The signs and symptoms describe the problem, not the etiology. NANDA (1989) suggests signs and symptoms associated with specific nursing diagnoses under the headings: defining characteristics. The characteristics are grouped according to frequency of occurrence. *Critical defining characteristics* must be present for the diagnosis to be made. *Major defining characteristics* appear to be present in all clients experiencing the problem. *Minor defining characteristics* are present in many clients experiencing the problem (NANDA, 1989, p. 560). Demonstrating the presence of the critical and major defining characteristics greatly increases the accuracy of the nursing diagnosis. This may be very helpful to the beginning student although practicing professional nurses do not often use this longer format.

The following would be examples of the same actual nursing diagnoses as above written in the PES format:

1. Impaired skin integrity related to immobility as manifested by disruption of the skin surface over the elbows and coccyx.
2. Parental role conflict related to divorce as manifested by statements of unsatisfactory child care during working hours.
3. Impaired verbal communication related to cultural differences as manifested by inability to speak English.

Potential Nursing Diagnoses. For a *potential nursing diagnosis* the nurse uses the following format:

$$\text{Potential Nursing Diagnosis} = \text{Problem} + \text{Risk Factors}$$

When making a potential nursing diagnosis the nurse is unable to list the signs and symptoms because the problem has not yet developed and, in fact, the nurse will attempt to intervene so the problem does not occur. Here the nurse lists the risk factors which have been identified from the assessment which indicate the problem is very likely to occur. The following are examples of potential nursing diagnoses:

Potential Nursing Diagnoses		
Problem	+	*Risk Factor*
1. Potential skin breakdown	r/t	physical immobilization in total body cast
2. Potential fluid volume deficit	r/t	diarrhea, age 3 yrs, low oral intake, elevated temperature
3. Potential for injury	r/t	disorientation and decreased vision after (cataract) surgery

Possible Nursing Diagnoses Finally, the nurse may write a *possible nursing diagnosis*. Because the purpose of this diagnosis is to assure continued data collection, it is not appropriate at this stage to identify either signs or symptoms or risk factors. The nurse would merely state:

Possible sensory-perceptual alteration
Possible nutritional deficit
Possible fluid volume deficit.

Each of these diagnoses requires that the nurse continue to collect sufficient data to make a decision regarding the existence of a nursing problem in this area.

The nurse is now ready to begin writing nursing diagnoses. The following steps summarize the process:

1. Review the assessment data.
2. Identify the problem focus area.
3. Consult NANDA listing of nursing diagnoses to aid in stating the problem.
4. State the cause if known.
5. State the signs, symptoms, risk factors if appropriate.

Occasionally the student will describe a problem that is not included in the NANDA listing. This may reflect an accurate problem. Nursing is an evolving science and the listing of nursing diagnoses is in the process of development. When this happens the nurse states the problem as clearly and as concisely as possible in a way that communicates the problem to those involved in the care of the patient. The nurse may wish to inform NANDA of this finding and follow the procedure for submitting a new diagnosis for approval and clinical testing.

SUMMARY

The process of making a nursing diagnosis consists of three activities: data analysis, problem identification, and the formulation of nursing diagnoses. During data analysis the nurse makes decisions based on the data regarding the health status of the patient. Next the nurse identifies problem focus areas and finally states a nursing diagnosis. The nursing diagnosis includes the patient problem and cause or etiology if known. The statement may also include signs and symptoms if the student is using the PES format. If it is a potential nursing diagnosis, the nurse includes the identification of risk factors which determined the diagnosis.

PRACTICE EXERCISE

Pick out the correctly written nursing diagnoses. Identify what is wrong with the incorrectly written nursing diagnoses. (Either the abbreviated formula or the PES formula is acceptable.) The correct answers follow the exercise.

1. Alteration in nutrition: less than body requirements related to nausea following chemotherapy.
2. Range of motion exercises (ROM) following a cerebral vascular accident (CVA).
3. Cancer of the breast with metastasis to the axillary lymph nodes.
4. Refusing wound irrigation related to pain of procedure.
5. Body image disturbance related to amputation of right foot.
6. Potential for sexual dysfunction in relating to husband and friends related to mastectomy.
7. Intermittent positive pressure breathing (IPPB) exercises q.i.d. to increase lung expansion
8. Pain and fear related to surgical procedure.
9. Severe itching related to a fungal infection.
10. Activity intolerance related to shortness of breath on activity.
11. Impaired physical mobility associated with right sided paralysis.
12. Ineffective breathing pattern etiology unknown, as evidenced by shortness of breath, tachypnea, pursed lip breathing.
13. Disorientation to time and place related to confused state.
14. Impaired verbal communication related to inability to speak dominant English language.
15. Fear related to uncertain outcome of surgery as manifested by urinary frequency, irritability, rapid pulse, ''It's all I can think about—I'm sure it's cancer.''
16. Ambulate progressively with tripod cane.
17. Potential for infection related to second degree burns on right hand.
18. Patient is upset and worried about the cost of hospitalization.
19. Impaired skin integrity related to prolonged bed rest as manifested by skin breakdown over both elbows and coccyx.
20. Thrombophlebitis related to prolonged bed rest as manifested by a positive Homan's sign.

ANSWERS TO EXERCISE ON NURSING DIAGNOSIS

1. Correct.   *Problem* = less than body requirements for nutritional needs.
   Cause   = nausea following chemotherapy.
   In this case nursing care will focus on methods to relieve the nausea.
2. Incorrect.
   Range of motion exercises are a nursing action.

3. Incorrect.
   Cancer of the breast is a medical diagnosis which the nurse is not licensed to treat. The experienced nurse might anticipate possible nursing diagnoses having to do with pain, body image, fear, or anxiety.

4. Incorrect.
   This is a nursing problem. The real nursing diagnosis may be something like: Pain associated with irrigation procedure. There would be many things the nurse could do to deal with the pain and make the procedure more acceptable to the patient.

5. Correct.   *Problem* = body image disturbance
                Cause   = amputation of the right foot

6. Correct.   *Problem* = potential for sexual dysfunction
                Cause   = related to mastectomy

7. Incorrect. This is a medical treatment.

8. Incorrect. These are two separate problems which will each require different nursing care.

9. Correct.   *Problem* = severe itching
                Cause   = fungal infection
   While this diagnosis is not listed in a NANDA format it does clearly convey the patient problem. However, the nurse does need additional information regarding the location of the infection. In this case the PES format would be helpful. In the NANDA format this nursing diagnosis might read: Alteration in comfort: pruritus related to fungal infection as manifested by patient complaints, scratch marks and rash on right leg, restlessness.

10. Incorrect. SOB is not a cause but a sign/symptom. Need etiology if known in diagnostic statement.

11. Correct.

12. Correct. P = ineffective breathing pattern
                E = unknown
                S = shortness of breath, tachypnea, pursed-lip breathing

13. Incorrect. Problem and cause are the same.

14. Correct.   *Problem* = impaired verbal communication
                Cause   = inability to speak dominant English language.

15. Correct. P = anxiety
                E = uncertain outcome of surgery
                S = urinary frequency, irritability, rapid pulse, "It's all I can think about—I'm sure it's cancer."

16. Incorrect. This is a physician's order.

17. Correct. *Problem* = potential for infection

Cause = related to second degree burns on right hand

18. Incorrect. This is a judgment. It may indicate that there is a problem but additional data is needed. This may be a problem that the nurse will refer to a social worker who has additional resources to assist this patient.

19. Correct. *P* = impaired skin integrity

E = related to prolonged bed rest

S = skin breakdown over coccyx and both elbows

20. Incorrect. This is a medical diagnosis, but it would suggest possible nursing diagnoses related to physical safety and pain. These would need further patient data for confirmation.

CASE STUDY: NURSING DIAGNOSES

The case study of Mrs. Witten is continued from Chapter 1 to identify nursing diagnoses. The NANDA approved diagnostic categories are used. Two different formats are used for stating the diagnosis of an actual problem. The first format uses the three parts: problem identification, etiology, and signs and symptoms of the problem (PES format). The second format uses two parts: problem identification and etiology. The signs and symptoms are listed under the category of "supporting data."

Mrs. Witten: Nursing Diagnoses

Example 1.

a. Pain secondary to possible gallbladder disease as evidenced by verbal report of RUQ pain, restlessness, elevated pulse and respirations.

b. Pain secondary to possible gallbladder disease

supporting data: c/o acute pain in RUQ; pulse 95, respirations 28, restless and clenching hands, gritting teeth, admitting medical diagnosis is to rule out cholecystitis

Example 2.

a. Fear related to illness and possible surgery as evidenced by report of being "scared," elevated pulse and respirations, crying, and muscle tension.

   b. Fear related to illness and possible surgery.

        supporting data: reports feeling ''scared''; states never been hospitalized; tears in eyes; pulse 96; diaphoretic (sweating); respirations 28; trembling hands.

Example 3.

   a. Altered health maintenance related to lack of knowledge and skill in breast self exam (BSE) as evidenced by statement of not doing BSE because it was never learned.

   b. Altered health maintenance related to lack of knowledge and skill in BSE.

        supporting data: reports she does not do BSE; states ''never learned.''

CHAPTER 3

Planning

III. The plan of nursing care includes goals derived from the nursing diagnoses.

IV. The plan of nursing care includes the priorities and the prescribed nursing approaches or measures to achieve the goals derived from the nursing diagnoses. (Standards of Nursing Practice, American Nurses' Association, 1973)

Now that the nurse has collected data about a patient, analyzed that data, and formulated some nursing diagnoses, the planning phase of the nursing process begins. In the planning phase, the nurse develops a plan to assist the patient to an optimum or improved level of functioning in the problem areas identified in the nursing diagnoses. The nurse analyzes the strengths and weaknesses of the patient, the patient's family, the nursing personnel, the health care facility, and the available resources (including other health professionals). The nurse also examines personal strengths, beliefs, and values that might affect the care planning phase. A nurse who is unable or unwilling to work with a patient in a particular problem area may need to seek help from another more experienced staff nurse, clinical instructor, or other resource.

A plan is developed to make nursing care both individualized for the patient and realistic for the hospital or home care setting. The skills of problem solving and decision making are applied to a particular patient's identified problems. The resulting plan of nursing care is designed to help patients and their families:

—maintain their current level of health and functioning if they are identified at risk for developing problems

A nurse remembers confronting personal limitations . . .

. . . . . *I remember the first time I was assigned to work with a newborn having a cleft lip and palate. Intellectually, I knew the baby needed special help with feeding and that this problem was fairly well correctable with surgery. I knew the mother was going through a grief process and had refused to hold her baby, and I thought to myself that the mother was very uncaring and I was even a little angry with her for acting this way. This all occurred to me during change of shift report; I had never actually seen a baby with a cleft lip and palate before. When I went into the nursery, the sight of that baby up close made me physically gag! I was so upset with myself, but I knew, that day, I was unable to help either the baby or the mother the way they deserved to be cared for. My head nurse understood and reassigned me without any criticism. I was full of self-incrimination thinking I would never become a good nurse. After a few days of watching other more experienced nurses care for, talk to and cuddle that baby, I was able to begin to see past the defect. I was so grateful to that head nurse for understanding and reassuring me that I'd get over my initial feelings. I also learned not to be so quick to condemn patient's responses to situations but to give them time to adjust.*

—reach an improved level of health and functioning
—adjust to reduced level of health and functioning when improvement is not possible
—adjust to a progressively decreasing level of functioning when terminally ill.

There are three steps in the planning phase: setting priorities among the nursing diagnoses when a patient has several problems, establishing goals with a patient, and planning specific nursing interventions to help a patient achieve the goals.

$$\text{Planning} = \frac{\text{Setting}}{\text{Priorities}} + \frac{\text{Establishing}}{\text{Goals}} + \frac{\text{Planning}}{\text{Nursing Interventions}}$$

SETTING PRIORITIES

During the process of priority setting, the nurse and the patient, whenever possible, mutually determine which problems identified during the assessment phase are in need of immediate attention and which problems might be dealt with at a later time. Consider assigning identified patient problems a high, middle, or low priority. The higher priority problems deserve the most immediate nursing attention for a plan and treatment. Setting priorities serves the purpose of ordering the delivery of nursing care so that more important or life threatening problems are treated before less critical problems. Priority setting does not mean that one problem must be totally resolved before another problem is considered. Problems can frequently be approached simultaneously. At times, decreasing the severity of one problem works to eliminate the others, as when eliminating severe pain corrects an ineffective breathing pattern.

Guidelines for Setting Priorities

1. Maslow's hierarchy of basic needs can guide the selection of high-priority problems. Survival needs that are significantly unmet pose the greatest threat to life and functioning and thus deserve a high priority rating. Using Maslow's theory to guide the delivery of nursing care, the nurse would:
    —Relieve a patient's pain (physiological need) before encouraging morning hygiene (self-esteem).
    —Encourage a new mother to express her disappointment about having a C-section when she had planned on totally natural childbirth (self-esteem) before teaching her infant care skills (self-actualization)
    —Stabilize bleeding and ensure adequate oxygenation in an emergency room accident victim before assessing elimination status (both of these are basic physiological needs, but oxygenation is usually the highest priority need; bleeding is considered a threat to tissue oxygenation)
    —Consider how difficult it is for you to read and absorb the material in this book (self-actualization need) if you have had too little sleep (physiological need)
    Basic survival needs will usually take priority over higher-level needs if the survival needs are not being satisfied. This is the case when a patient is in obvious physical distress owing to the unmet need. If the survival needs are being partially met and actual physical distress is tolerable, a higher-level need may take priority or at least have the same priority as a lower-level need. For example, an auto accident victim can be in considerable distress with multiple physical needs unmet, yet the priority need may be to ascertain the whereabouts and injuries of the other

family members in the car when it crashed. This unmet higher-level need can have a negative effect on satisfaction of this patient's physical needs if it is not given appropriate attention.

2. Focus on the problems the patient feels are most important if this priority does not interfere with medical treatment. A patient's need for undisturbed rest cannot take precedence over a medically ordered treatment for observation of blood pressure and pulse every hour following a car accident.

    If there are no nursing contraindications, offer patients the opportunity to set their own priorities. However, do not offer patients the opportunity to make choices they really do not have, or are not qualified to make. After surgery, the patient and family may identify the need for rest and pain management as priority concerns, while the nurse is equally concerned about maintaining a clear airway and improving gas exchange based on an assess-

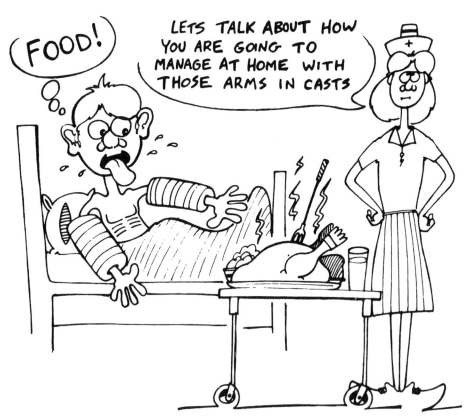

FIGURE 3-1. Priority setting.

ment of diminished breath sounds and moist gurgling heard in the lungs. The challenge for the nurse is to help all involved understand and agree about which problems will be dealt with now, and which problems may have to wait until the patient is more stable.

Mutual priority setting with the patient serves two purposes. First, this approach involves patients in planning their own care. Perhaps the nurse has overlooked a major problem that is consuming the patient's time and energy or has assigned the problem a low priority. Unless this problem is considered first, the nurse may be able to achieve only limited success in other areas because the patient is still worrying about the overlooked problem. Second, cooperation between the nurse and the patient is enhanced when priority setting is done together. The nurse often acts as an interpreter by stating recognition of the patient and family concerns, sharing nursing and medical concerns with the patient/family, and guiding priority setting to promote safe physical care, attend to patient's concerns as soon as possible, and fit within the time and work constraints of the health care setting. The nurse also identifies patient/family concerns to the physician, other nurses, and other health professionals who may then reset their priorities based on a better understanding of the patient's status.

3. Consider the effect of potential problems when setting priorities. For example:

   —A new mother may ask to be left alone with her husband and newborn to get acquainted. The potential problem of a postpartum hemorrhage developing would require continuous observation after delivery, since this is potentially life threatening. Thus the patient's request to be left alone cannot be safely met.

   —A bedridden patient may be started on a routine of frequent turning and positioning to prevent bed sores and contractures, even though the patient may not see this as important. Prevention of the potential complications of prolonged bedrest is a high priority, since treating these problems after they develop is less effective, more costly, and usually more time consuming than preventive measures.

   Prevention of a potential problem, rather than treatment of the problem when it develops, is a goal deserving continuous assessment and intervention.

4. Consider costs, resources available, personnel, and time needed

to plan for and treat each of the patient's identified problems. If resources, personnel, time, or financing is currently unavailable to deal with a particular problem, it may receive a low priority until some of these obstacles have been overcome. If a problem can be quickly resolved, it may receive a high priority for practical reasons.

5. Consider state laws, hospital policy statements, and outcome criteria established for the particular setting. For example, in many states it is the law that all children under the age of 4 years must be transported in an approved car seat. Hospital policy may state that newborns must be taken home by their parents in an appropriate car seat. This potential problem of injury to the newborn if not in a car seat during an automobile accident should be discussed early to give the family time to obtain a car seat before discharge.

ESTABLISHING GOALS

The second step in the planning phase of the nursing process is to establish a goal for each of the patient's problems identified in the nursing diagnoses. A goal for an *actual nursing diagnosis* describes a change in the patient's health status or functioning: the desired outcome of nursing interventions. A goal can be thought of as an achievement, by the patient, which shows a reduction or lessening of the problem diagnosed by the nurse. For a *potential nursing diagnosis,* the goal is often to maintain the current problem-free status or current level of functioning.

NURSING GOAL:

The desired outcome of nursing care; that which you hope to achieve with your patient and which is designed to prevent, remedy, or lessen the problem identified in the nursing diagnosis.

Why Is A Goal Statement Needed?

A goal is needed as part of the plan of care because it gives guidance in the selection of nursing interventions. A goal is a constant reminder of why the nurse is doing certain activities with each patient. Goals give a standard against which to compare patient's hourly, daily, weekly, monthly, yearly, and lifelong efforts to maintain and improve health and functioning. Goals give a sense of where this particular patient started from and where the individual and the nurse hope to end up. The assessment data provide the *baseline* for the patient's current level of function in a problem area. For example, a newly diagnosed diabetic who has lost 20 pounds, is dehydrated, and is inadequately nourished. The goal might be for the individual to regain 15 lbs over the next two months, taking his prescribed amount of insulin each day. Progress toward this goal over the weeks will be measured against the original baseline data and the optimal weight gain identified in the goal statement. The goals nurses write will be the criteria used to evaluate the success of nursing interventions. A goal helps to motivate both the nurse and the patient to continue their efforts. When goals are achieved, it provides the patient, the patient's family, and the nurse and other caregivers with the reward of success, and success promotes further efforts to achieve other goals.

The goal for a student in nursing might be to graduate from school with a GPA of 3.0. Another student might set a higher or lower goal depending on competing life responsibilities and personal abilities. The same is true in nursing practice. Without a clear, concise goal statement, the nurse and the patient do not know if and when the desired end has been achieved.

The professional nurse is expected to demonstrate the ability to develop and communicate goals as part of each patient's care. The Joint Commission of Accreditation of Healthcare Organization (JCAHO), which is the national organization for accrediting hospitals, identifies, as one of their standards for approving a hospital, "Individualized, goal-directed nursing care is provided to patients through the use of the nursing process," (JCAHO, 1989).

Components of a Goal Statement

At least one goal is written for each nursing diagnosis. Sometimes several goals are written for one diagnosis, especially if there is a broad scope to the problem. Most goals are written to include specific components which are identified in the formula below.

$$\text{Goal Statement} = \text{Patient Behavior} + \text{Criteria of Performance} + \text{Time} + \text{Conditions (if Needed)}$$

Patient Behavior. The patient behavior the nurse selects for the goal statement is an observable activity that the patient will demonstrate. The activity can be seen, heard, felt, or measured by the nurse. The activity shows an improved level of functioning in the area identified by an actual nursing diagnosis. The activity may reflect maintenance of a current level of functioning in the problem area identified by a potential nursing diagnosis. The activity selected for the goal does not usually show a lessening or elimination of the cause (etiology) of the problem but focuses on the problem and what the patient will be able to do. The word "patient" or the patient's actual name may be omitted when writing the goal, since the goal always refers to the patient.

PATIENT BEHAVIOR = an observable activity that the patient will demonstrate

- —(the patient) will void
- —decrease in (the patient's) blood pressure
- —(the patient) will ambulate
- —(the patient) will report
- —(the patient) will drink

Criteria of Performance. The criteria of performance is a stated level or standard of the patient behavior selected for the goal. This part of the goal specifies a realistic improvement in functioning, by a stated time, to be used to judge or decide if the goal was satisfactorily achieved. The criteria clarifies and individualizes the goal based on patients' current abilities and realistic expectations of their level of functioning in the future. If the identified behavior is to pass the course Nsg 101, is a grade of "D" an acceptable criterion for passing or should the minimum criterion be set at the "C" level? Some goals identify the optimum level of recovery (optimum criteria) or functioning for a patient after treatment, and often span weeks or months. These are described as long-term goals. Other goals identify lesser changes in patient behavior and may span minutes to days. These are short-term goals.

CRITERIA OF ACCEPTABLE PERFORMANCE = the level at which the patient will perform the behavior. How well? How long? How far? How much?

- —at least 500 ml of urine
- —below the value of 160/100 mmHg

—the length of the hall, three times
—a level of 4 or less (on a 1-10 scale)
—1500 ml of liquid intake

Time Frame. The goal statement includes a time or date to clarify how long it would realistically take for the patient to reach the level of functioning stated in the criteria part of the goal. This is based on nursing knowledge, experience, and constraints of the health care setting. The time stated in the goal may be minutes, hours, days, weeks, or months.

TIME = the designated time or date when the patient should be able to achieve the behavior. A long-term goal attempts to identify how long it will take a patient to achieve the optimal recovery of functioning.

—within the next hour
—by discharge
—at the end of this shift
—by June 5
—in 2 months

Conditions. Sometimes the nurse sets goals with the patient that require the use or presence of certain environmental conditions. Conditions can be thought of as specific aides which will facilitate the patient performing a behavior at the level in the criteria and within the specified time frame.

CONDITION = the circumstances, if important, under which the behavior will be performed. All goals will not have a condition. If the condition is important, put it in the goal statement; if it is not important, leave it out.

—with the help of a walker
—with the use of a wheelchair
—with the help of the family
—with the use of medication
—using IM Demerol q3–4 hrs
—using oral analgesics q3–4 hrs
—without analgesics
—on twice daily insulin injections

The following examples combine these elements to form goal statements.

Goal Statements

Patient Behavior	+ Criteria	+ Time	+ Condition (if relevant)
Weight gain	of ½ ounce	every day until discharge	on 24 calorie/oz formula.
Weight gain	of ¼ ounce	every day until discharge	on breast-feeding with no supplement.
Self-injection	of correct insulin dose, using sterile technique	by November 4	using an autoinjector.
Maintenance of joint mobility	at current level	while on bedrest.	
Regain	15 lbs	in 2 months	on 2300 cal. diet and twice daily insulin injections.
Oral intake	of 500 ml	by 3 P.M.	without abdominal distention, nausea or vomiting.
Report pain reduced	at a level of 4 or less	during the first 24° postop	with Demerol 50–100 mg IM q3–4 hrs, prn
Report pain reduced	at a level of 4 or less	during 24°–48° postop	with the use of oral analgesics q3–4 hrs, prn
Will void	at least 300 cc	before bladder becomes distended.	
Will void	at least 200 cc	within 6 hours	after removal of Foley catheter.

Long- and Short-Term Goals

All goals include a time at which point the patient is to be evaluated for goal achievement. Goals can be classified as short- and long-term goals based on the length of time the patient is expected to take to accomplish the behavior identified in the goal. The nurse may believe that some goals are so critical to patient survival that goal achievement is set in terms of hours or less. Other goals dealing with optimum recovery from health problems may span weeks to years.

This is like an examination schedule in education. By mid-quarter time, you should know objectives 1–10 and by final exam you will be tested on the entire course content. Longer-term goals tend to have higher expectations for level of functioning based on improvement or learning over time. By discharge from the hospital in three days, the patient might be expected to achieve a certain improved level of functioning compared to current levels. By a four week check-up visit, the patient might be expected to be at a higher level. Both the differing behavioral expectations and the time frame go into classifying goals as long or short term.

Short-Term Goals. Short-term goals identify outcomes in patients' status or behavior that can be achieved fairly quickly, in a matter of hours or days. Short-term goals are especially appropriate to acute-care settings, such as intensive care units, emergency rooms, recovery rooms, to name a few. Patients in these settings are unstable, and their physical status is often changing rapidly. The long-term prognosis for these patients is uncertain, and health care is focused on the present.

If a problem is diagnosed that tends to worsen with the passage of time, in terms of hours or days short-term goals are more appropriate than long-term goals. The nurse wants to see a change in patient behavior soon; the problem cannot be allowed to continue until physical or psychological damage occurs. For example, the patient who is unable to void following surgery cannot be left for 24 hours with a filling bladder. Extreme discomfort and possible damage to the bladder or kidneys could be the consequence. A short-term goal is identified for a patient following surgery, such as "reestablishment of urinary elimination within 6 to 8 hours after surgery." If the patient is unable to achieve this goal, a catheter is often inserted to empty the bladder and prevent damage. Not all short-term goals are written on a patient's plan of care. Setting goals is a way of thinking. Rather than thinking of separate tasks to accomplish this shift, such as bed bath, V.S. R.O.M. exercises, and meds, the nurse thinks "What can I realistically accomplish with this patient in the next few hours to help lessen or eliminate the diagnosed problem?"

Some examples of short-term goals are the following:

Respirations below 30 breaths/minute within 1 hour.
Return of bowel sounds within 12 hours postop.
Passing flatus within 24 hours postop.
Temperature to be below 102°F within 1 hour.
Pain to be rated as 4 or less within 30 minutes.
For the reader of this book: Completion of Chapter 2 in the next hour.

When learning to write goals, start with short-term goals. A beginning nursing student is not with the same patient for long periods of time.

Students may care for a patient for only a few hours. By writing a short-term goal involving the length of time with the patient, the student will be able to give the needed nursing care and evaluate the results. By evaluating whether the goal was met before leaving the patient, students will gain skill in writing realistic goals and in giving nursing care to meet those goals.

Short-term goals are often developed to help the nurse and the patient gauge progress toward long-term goals. By achieving short-term goals, the patient is gradually advanced to the improved or optimum level of functioning identified in the long-term goal. Achievement of short-term goals provides repeated satisfaction for both the nurse and the patient, serving as evidence of progress and guidance for the future. For example, the nurse and the patient have identified a long-term goal, ''weight loss of 80 pounds in 1 year.'' Progressive short-term goals are identified to help the nurse and the patient measure progress toward long-term goal achievement. For example,

Weight of 210 pounds by February 7
Weight of 208 pounds by February 14
Weight of 206 pounds by February 21

A series of short-term goals that a person can realistically accomplish in a stated time period is much more rewarding than striving for one long-term goal. The repeated reinforcement a person receives from meeting short-term goals can keep an individual motivated to achieve a long-term goal. If short-term goals are not achieved, new nursing interventions can be tried, more realistic goals can be selected, or the nurse may reanalyze the data and diagnosis to make sure the problem is accurately identified, and important to the patient.

Some other examples of short-term goals leading to a long-term goal are the following:

1. ''I will finish reading this book before final exams'' might be a long-term goal for a student in nursing. This student might accomplish the long-term goal by progressive short-term goals of reading one chapter each week.
2. ''Patient will demonstrate full use of broken arm within 6 months.'' This patient might accomplish the long-term goal by progressively increasing the amount and range of muscle/joint exercises.
3. ''Performance of self-care activities within 3 months of cerebral vascular accident (stroke).'' Progressive short-term goals might

focus on accomplishment of one self-care activity a week until the patient was able to perform many activities independently.

Week of 10/10: Feeds self by end of week.

Week of 10/17: Brushing teeth by end of week.

Week of 10/24: Performs personal hygiene by end of week.

Week of 10/31: Meets own mobility needs by end of week.

Long-Term Goals.   Long-term goals give direction for nursing care over time. Long-term goals can be thought of as an eventual destination while progressive short-term goals are a series of stops on the way to the final destination. This is similar to planning a car trip. You want to be in Florida by March 28th. To achieve that long-term goal, you must be in Chicago by March 25th, and in Georgia by March 27th. Long-term goals try to identify the maximum level of functioning possible for a patient with a particular nursing diagnosis. Consider the prognosis of the patient's health problems, resources available, strengths and weakness of the patient and family, and nursing care abilities of personnel who will be working with the patient. If the patient has an alteration in some function, the long-term goal is to restore a normal pattern of functioning, if possible. If that is not possible, the goal deals with establishing a maximum level of functioning for the alteration and assisting the patient to adjust to this altered level of functioning. Some examples of long-term goals are the following:

Reestablishment of patient's usual bowel elimination patterns in 2 months.

Reestablish normal voiding patterns by 5 days postop.

Breastfeeding 10 to 15 minutes/breast, every 2 to 5 hours, within 2 weeks of delivery.

Self-care of colostomy 1 month after surgery.

Patient to state no longer afraid of having severe pain during terminal illness from cancer after 1 week on IV morphine pump.

For the reader of this book: Utilization of the nursing process to assess, diagnose, plan, implement, and evaluate the care of patients, following graduation from a school of nursing.

Some goals are designed to maintain a continuous level of functioning during the time the patient is receiving nursing care. These goals are usually related to potential rather than actual nursing diagnoses. They do not have a specified time for goal achievement but rather imply systematic assessment and evaluation for as long as the problem exists. These goals are considered long-term goals and span several days to weeks or more. For example:

1. Patient to report pain management techniques are adequate during hospitalization.
2. Patient to report pain remains below 4 on a 1–10 scale during the postoperative period.
3. Skin integrity maintained during hospitalization.
4. Normal breath sounds maintained during postoperative period.
5. Maintenance of body weight between 135 and 140 pounds (forever).

These goals would be evaluated periodically as part of the plan of care rather than having a set time or date for evaluation as with other goals discussed. For example (see goals above):

1. Assess pain every 3 to 4 hours
2. Assess pain on 1–10 scale every 3 to 4 hours
3. Assess skin integrity every 2 hours
4. Assess breath sounds every 4 hours
5. Assess body weight every morning

These assessments would then be documented in the patient's chart until the potential for the problem was eliminated.

Guidelines for Writing Goal Statements

From JCAHO's *Accreditation Manual for Hospitals* comes the required activities for hospital registered nurses: "A registered nurse plans each patient's nursing care."

—Whenever possible, nursing goals are mutually set with the patient and/or the family.
—Nursing goals are based on the nursing assessment and are realistic, measurable, and consistent with the therapy prescribed by the responsible medical practioner. (JCAHO, 1989)

When learning to write goal statements for nursing diagnoses, make sure long- and short-term goals meet the following criteria:

1. **For an actual nursing diagnosis, the goal statement is a patient behavior that demonstrates reduction or alleviation of the problem.** Start with the nursing diagnosis. What is the

problem? If the nursing diagnosis is "Pain related to broken right arm as evidenced by patient report, crying and elevated pulse," the goal will demonstrate alleviation or lessening of the pain (not healing of the arm). If the nursing diagnosis is "Constipation related to dehydration and use of analgesics with codeine," the goal deals with bowel elimination patterns showing restoration of normal function (not improved hydration or limiting the amount of codeine). The following examples in Table 3-1 demonstrate the relationship between the nursing diagnosis and the goal statement. A general nursing diagnostic category from the NANDA list is presented first, with individualized diagnostic statements underneath. Two formats are used for the diagnostic statement of actual nursing diagnoses, the three part statement and the two part statement with supporting data underneath. A long-term goal and one or more short-term goals are identified for each diagnosis.

Table 3–1   Relationship of the Diagnosis to the Goals

Nursing Diagnoses	*Goal Statements*
Alteration in bowel elimination:	Reestablish normal bowel pattern by discharge
○ *constipation related to dehydration and bedrest as evidenced by hard to pass stool and no BM for 5 days	○ bowel movement by 3 P.M. today following Fleets enema
○ constipation related to dehydration and bedrest supporting data: no BM for 5 days; reports stool hard to pass	○ bowel movement tomorrow without use of enema
Alteration in comfort:	Report of negligible pain by discharge
○ *pain related to tissue trauma secondary to surgery as evidenced by rating pain as 8, elevated pulse and BP 136/72	○ pain reported at a level of 3 or less within the next hour
○ pain related to tissue trauma secondary to surgery supporting data: pulse 92, BP 136/72 pain rated as 8	○ pain reduced to a level of 3 or less during the next 24 hours with IM analgesics ○ pain reduced to a level of 3 or less after 48 hours postop with oral analgesic

Table 3–1   Relationship of the Diagnosis to the Goals (*Cont.*)

Nursing Diagnoses	Goal Statements
Ineffective airway clearance	Independent maintenance of clear airway by 3/8.
◦ *ineffective airway clearance related to weakness and lowered level of consciousness as evidenced by inability to remove secretions from back of throat ◦ ineffective airway clearance related to weakness and lowered LOC. supporting data: generalized weakness; gurgling of mucus in throat; difficult to arouse; 86 years old; 1 hr postop	◦ airway free of tracheal mucus within the next ½ hour ◦ productive cough by 12 hours ◦ clear breath sounds in 24 hours

* = PES format (problem + etiology + signs/symptoms)

2. **For potential nursing diagnoses, the goal statement is a patient behavior that demonstrates maintenance of the current status of health or functioning.** If the potential nursing diagnosis is "Potential for impaired skin integrity related to casting of left leg," the goal will demonstrate maintenance of intact skin (not healing of the leg). If the nursing diagnosis is "Potential for ineffective thermoregulation related to newborn status," the goal demonstrates maintenance of the newborn's temperature in the normal range.

3. **The goal is realistic for the patient's capabilities in the time span you designate in your goal.** A goal for a preterm baby weighing 4 pounds, that stated, "Baby will weigh 8 pounds at the end of 1 week," would be unrealistic for this newborn. But if the goal stated, "Baby will weigh 4½ pounds in 7 days," the capabilities of the patient have been considered and make the goal more realistic and more likely to be achieved. Experience, professional literature, references, and advice from other more experienced nurses will help the student learn what is realistic for patients with particular problems.

4. **The goal is realistic for the nurse's level of skill and experience.** If the nursing diagnosis is dealing with a problem beyond

the nurse's role, the best course of action is to refer the problem to the appropriate professional. A patient with a nursing diagnosis of "Alteration in nutrition: less than body requirements related to refusal to eat hospital food as evidenced by 5 lb weight loss" is referred to a dietitian. A patient with a nursing diagnosis of "Impaired verbal communication related to recent stroke as evidenced by inability to say any word except 'no,' " is referred to a speech therapist when the patient's condition is sufficiently stable.

5. **The goal is congruent with and supportive of other therapies.** This means that nursing goals for the patient do not contradict or interfere with the work of other professionals caring for the patient. If the nursing diagnosis is "Urinary retention related to decreased urge, and perineal swelling as evidenced by residual urine volumes over 500 cc $\times 2$," a goal to have the patient void 300 cc this shift would be in conflict with a medical order to leave the catheter in place for 12 hours if the second residual urine was more than 200 cc.

6. **Whenever possible the goal is important and valued by the patient, the nurses, and the physician.** If goals are important to patients, they will be more motivated to reach them. If nurses value the goal, they will be more likely to carry out the suggested plan of care. The physician's understanding and support of nursing goals will help to assure congruence with medical treatment. The goals also serve as a communication tool that keeps health team members informed of the patient's progress.

7. **The goal is an observable or measurable patient behavior.** This means the nurse can see, hear, feel, or measure the patient's response. Try to avoid words such as good, normal, adequate, and improved. These words mean different things to different people and tend to make the goal unclear. There may be disagreement as to whether the goal was achieved if words requiring a judgment are used in the goal statement. Remember, the nurse cannot see a patient "understanding," "feeling," or "knowing about."

Observable verbs

reports	eats	sleeps
walks	drinks	breathes
rates	voids	demonstrates

Observable Goals	*Vague Goals*
The patient will walk the length of the hall unassisted by 2/5.	Increased ambulation or adequate leg strength
Patient will gain 1/4 lb each week until discharged.	Increased intake or good nutrition or promote weight gain

8. **Write goals in terms of patient outcomes, not nursing actions.**

Patient Outcomes	*Nursing Actions*
The patient will void by 6 P.M.	I will offer the patient the urinal every 2 hours.
The patient will safely bathe her baby before she is discharged.	I will show the patient a baby bath before she is discharged.
The patient's temperature will be up to 98°F within 1 hour.	I will put warm blankets and a heating pad on the patient and recheck his temperature in 1 hour.

9. **Keep the goal short.**
10. **Make the goal specific.**
11. **Derive each goal from only one nursing diagnosis.**
12. **Designate a specific time for achievement of each goal.**

Practice Exercise

Pick out the correctly written goal statements. Identify what is wrong with the incorrectly written goals. The answers follow the exercise.

1. The patient's hydration will improve.
2. The nurse will reduce the patient's anxiety.
3. The patient will know about infant feeding.
4. Improve muscle strength.
5. 3/5: The patient will lose 6 lb in 2 weeks.

6. The patient will talk about her labor within 24 hours after delivery.

7. The decubitus ulcer (bedsore) will be healed by 2/5.

8. Verbalization of decreased pain within the next hour.

9. The patient will express confidence in her ability to breastfeed her baby before discharge.

10. Turn and deep breathe the patient every 2 hours.

11. Ankle edema will decrease.

12. The patient will feel better by bedtime.

13. The patient will ambulate.

14. Teach the patient AROM (active range of motion) exercises.

15. The patient's depression will improve.

16. The patient will learn about good nutrition.

17. The patient will understand the purpose of his medications before discharge.

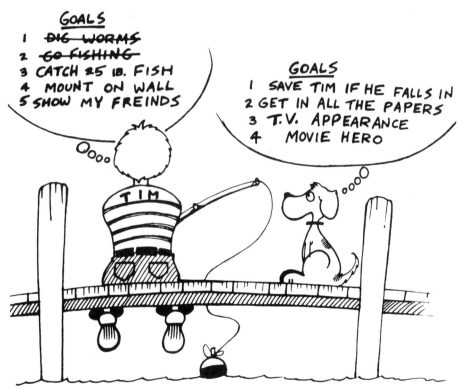

FIGURE 3–2. Goal setting.

18. The patient's temperature will stay below 101°F during the next 24 hours.
19. The nursing student will understand the nursing process after reading this book.
20. The student will write a nursing diagnosis and a goal after finishing this chapter.

Answers to Exercise on Goal Statements

1. Not specific or observable. A better goal would be:
    The patient's intake will be 2500 cc every 24 hours.
    or
    The patient will drink at least 75 cc each hour.
2. Not observable. This is a nurse behavior instead of patient behavior. No time limit is set. A better goal would be:
    Verbalization of reduced anxiety about tomorrow's surgery by 10 P.M. tonight.
    or
    The patient will discuss feelings related to biopsy by 3 P.M. today.
3. Not observable, no time limit. A better goal would be:
    (The patient) Feeding her baby the majority of his feedings by 6/7.
    or
    Newborn regained birth weight on breast milk by 2-week check-up.
4. No subject, not specific, no criteria. A better goal would be:
    The patient will lift his own weight using the bed trapeze by 2/5.
    or
    4/5: The patient will be able to lift equal amounts of weight in 3 months with his right and his left arm.
5. O.K.
6. O.K.
7. O.K.
8. O.K. Subject (the patient) is assumed.
9. O.K.
10. This is a nursing action, not an observable patient behavior.

11. Not specific, no time limit. A better goal would be:
     Absence of edema of the ankle by tomorrow at 10 P.M.
     or
     Ankle will measure 10 inches in circumference or less by to-
     morrow at 8 A.M.
12. Not observable. A better goal would be:
     The patient will state anxiety about being hospitalized has de-
     creased by H.S.
13. No criteria. A better goal would be:
     The patient will walk the length of the hall by date of discharge
     without use of a walker.
     or
     8/2: The patient will walk from his bed to a chair in his room
     by tomorrow.
14. Nursing action instead of patient behavior, no time limit. A bet-
     ter goal would be:
     The patient will demonstrate AROM by 3 P.M. today.
     or
     The patient will have equal motion in the right and left shoulder
     joint by time of discharge.
15. Too vague, not observable. A better goal would be:
     The patient will sit in patient lounge for 15 minutes during this
     shift.
     or
     8/3: The patient will get dressed and comb her hair tomorrow
     A.M.
16. Not observable. A better goal would be:
     (The patient) Select a food from each of the four basic food
     groups for tonight's supper.
     or
     (The patient) Plan a week's menu for a low-salt diet with the
     help of the dietitian before discharge.
17. Not observable. A better goal would be:
     The patient will state the purpose of each of his medications
     before discharge.
     or
     By 4/7, the patient will state route, dose, and time for each
     take-home medication.
18. O.K.
19. Not observable. A better goal would be:

The nursing student will list the steps in the nursing process after reading this book.
or
The nursing student will write one nursing care plan after reading this book.
   20.   O.K.

PLANNING NURSING INTERVENTIONS

Nursing interventions are activities the nurse plans and implements to help a patient achieve identified goals. By achieving these goals, the patient will reduce or eliminate the diagnosed problems. Nursing interventions may be referred to in several ways: nursing actions, nursing strategies, nursing treatment plans, and nursing orders. This text will use all these terms to mean the same things. Some texts use the term nursing interventions to mean a general activity, such as "force fluids" and a nursing action or order then refers to a specific, individualized activity, such as "100 cc fluids q2h $\times$ next 24°." The nurse, using a problem-solving approach, selects activities to do with and for the patient that are most likely to result in goal achievement. There are many nursing interventions to choose from to help reduce a given problem. The nurse tries to select the best ones, based on the desired goal, patient abilities and preferences, available resources, nursing knowledge and experience, and protocols of the health care facility.

The planned nursing interventions are communicated to other nurses on the patient care plan to promote a consistent approach toward goal achievement. Often the nurse who has the most information about the patient and expertise in the particular problem areas diagnosed is the one who selects the most appropriate nursing interventions. The written care plan communicates this plan for goal achievement to others who will provide 24-hour nursing care to the patient. The nursing interventions written on the patient's care plan are instructions for others to follow since they may not have the knowledge of, or experience with, the patient that the original nurse gained during the assessment phase.

Nursing interventions are similar to physician's orders since they specify a plan of care aimed at achieving a goal. In order for others to follow a plan of care, it must be specific or the plan may be interpreted inappropriately. Interventions should identify:

—what is to be done
—when the activity is to be done; how often

—the duration for each intervention, when appropriate

—any preceding or follow-up activities

—the date interventions were selected

—the sequence in which nursing activities are to be performed, when one activity is dependent on or facilitated by a previous action

—signature or initials of the nurse writing the plan of care

When these things are identified by the professional nurse on a patient's plan of nursing care, other nurses are held responsible and accountable to the patient, nurse colleagues, and the health care facility for the prescribed care. Other nurses know to whom to direct questions regarding the patient. They know to whom to direct feedback regarding patient responses following the prescribed care. Physicians may seek out the nurse who wrote the plan of care for a patient as the person most knowledgeable about that patient's response to ordered treatments. All of this may seem somewhat threatening to the student in nursing who may feel unsure of abilities to identify accurate diagnoses, select appropriate goals, and choose nursing interventions most likely to achieve those goals. It is a learning process, but without both positive and negative feedback from other nurses who carry out the plan, students will not improve skills in planning patient care.

NURSING INTERVENTIONS:

Those specific activities the nurse plans and implements in order to help the patient achieve a goal.

Types of Nursing Interventions

There are several broad categories of nursing interventions. Combining actions from several different groups is often the most effective plan. These groupings of nursing interventions include:

1. **Environmental management**—This aspect of nursing care involves establishing and maintaining a safe, therapeutic environment. A noisy, cluttered, stark environment is not the best atmosphere to promote rest and recovery. Attention to room order, opening and closing curtains for light, wall calendars showing the correct date, opening and reading mail, keeping the bed clean and straightened and the night stand accessible with needed per-

sonal articles are all activities that fall into this category. These activities may not require the expertise of a professional nurse but it may be nursing's responsibility to help with or delegate these activities. The patient and family may be uneasy in a health care setting where no one attends to environmental management.

"Very few people . . . have any idea of the exquisite cleanliness required in the sick room. . . . The well have a curious habit of forgetting that what is to them but a trifling inconvenience, to be patiently "put up" with, is to the sick a source of suffering, delayed recovery, if not actually hastening death. The well are scarcely ever more than eight hours, at most in the same room. Some change they can make, if only for a few minutes. . . . But the sick man who never leaves his bed, who can not change by any movement of his own his air, or his light, or his warmth; who can not obtain quiet; or get out of the smoke, or the dust; he is really poisoned or depressed by what is to you the merest trifle."   *p. 92*

Florence Nightingale *Notes On Nursing: What It Is and What It Is Not.* From an unabridged republication of the first American edition as published in 1860. (1969) New York: Dover Publications.

---

2. **Physician initiated and ordered interventions**—Based on the physician's diagnosis of the patient's health problems, orders to assess patient status, schedule tests, and provide treatments will be written by the physician in the patient's chart. The nurse is expected to implement these orders. Implementation of these orders is still considered part of nursing interventions because the nurse individualizes the way the order is carried out based on the patient's status at the time. The nurse often explains what is to be done and why. The nurse may give the patient some choices within the scope of implementing the order. The timing of the implementation is often adjusted or designated by the professional nurse to fit in with constraints on personnel within the health care setting while still providing safety for the patient and performance of the ordered activity. An example is IV therapy. The physician orders the type and amount of fluid to infuse and the rate. The nurse often does the venipuncture, sets up the IV system and keeps it running. The nurse assesses the patient response frequently and may discontinue the infusion if problems develop. The nurse may refer the problem to a specially trained IV nurse to reinitiate treatment. Based on other assessments of

the patient, the nurse may discuss with the physician if reinitiation of therapy is desired since the patient is drinking well with good bowel sounds.

3. **Nurse initiated and physician ordered interventions**—Based on the nurse's assessment of the patient, and identification of problems, the nurse may request help from the physician in treatment. The nurse is not licensed to order certain treatments but recognizes when they may be needed. The nurse is requesting an intervention from the physician to help reduce or treat the problem the nurse has identified. An order to catheterize a patient unable to void may be written after the nurse notifies the physician of the problem, supporting data and ineffective interventions implemented thus far.

    Another example of this type of intervention occurs when the nurse collaborates with the physician regarding an order already written. The nurse may have identified a change in patient status and is questioning whether an order should be implemented as written or whether the physician would like to change the order based on current patient status and needs. For example the physician may have written the order to begin clear liquids postoperatively and to discontinue the IV when the current bag has infused. The patient is experiencing a variation from the normal postop course and is unable to take any fluids, is nauseated and vomiting, and has an increased pulse. To discontinue the IV at this point would not be prudent without updating the physician on the patient's response postop. The nurse requests the physician's help, identifies the alteration in patient status, and requests clarification of the original order.

    The physician frequently writes orders to be implemented only if the need arises (prn orders). The nurse then identifies if the problem develops, adapts the interventions to the patient's status, implements the adapted order, and documents the patient's response. This is the case when the physician writes prn orders for different forms of analgesia in a dosage range on a patient. The nurse and the patient determine need for the medication, intensity of pain, and the nurse selects the medication and dose most likely to meet the patient's need for pain relief.

4. **Nurse initiated and ordered interventions**—These interventions are solely in the range of professional nursing. The nurse assesses the patient, makes a nursing diagnosis, selects interventions, and implements those interventions or delegates implementation to other nursing personnel.

Within this category are several forms of independent nursing interventions:

a. health teaching

b. health counseling to assist patients make informed choices

c. referrals to other nurses or health care professionals; transfer summaries to other stations, hospitals, or nursing homes; public health referrals; home health agency referrals.

d. specific nursing treatments to prevent problems or lessen current difficulties, such as ambulating, turning and repositioning, suctioning the airway, feedings, cleaning and dressing a wound, range of motion exercises

e. providing support, comfort, and encouragement

f. assessment of patient status or response to treatments ordered by nursing, by physicians, or other health professionals

g. assistance with problem-solving related to life-style changes, coping with health changes and medical treatments, setting priorities. Examples might include problem-solving with a new diabetic patient on how to fit blood glucose monitoring, insulin injections, and food intake into a job requiring frequent travel and eating in restaurants.

h. assistance with meeting basic needs/activities of daily living

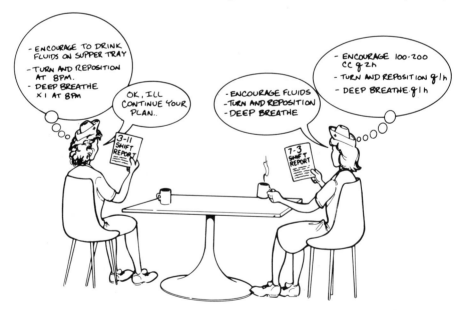

FIGURE 3–3. Care plans ensure continuity of care when written in specific rather than general terms.

Some examples of nursing interventions are the following:

SHORT-TERM GOAL: Reestablish urinary elimination, with complete emptying of the bladder within 6 hours of removal of catheter.

—Interventions:

1. Offer assistance to the bathroom for voiding every 2 hours
2. Encourage fluids, 1 glass of juice, every hour
3. Record intake and output for 24 hours
4. Offer analgesics every 3 to 4 hours
5. Provide privacy for voiding attempts
6. Run water in bathroom for voiding attempts
7. Encourage application of pressure over bladder during voiding attempts
8. Encourage voiding attempt in sitz bath, tub bath, or shower if unable to void in 5 hours
9. Assess bladder for emptying following voiding

Rationale for Nursing Interventions

Nursing actions are based on principles and knowledge integrated from previous nursing education and experience and from the behavioral and physical sciences. These principles identify the relationship between the nursing intervention and goal achievement. Nursing actions are known to affect people in predictable ways and are chosen to help a patient achieve a goal because of these expected outcomes. For example, the effects of heat and cold applied to the skin are understood by the nurse. If the nurse wants to increase the blood flow to an area of the body as one way of promoting goal achievement, a nursing intervention such as "warm packs to right arm, 20 minutes 4 times a day" might be chosen.

The first courses in many nursing programs involve the student in a study of basic fundamentals of nursing practice. These fundamentals courses provide the student with the rationale for the steps of various skills and procedures in addition to teaching the motor aspects of the skill or procedure. In order to safely adapt nursing care to new situations, new equipment, and changing technology, the nurse must understand the rationale behind the choice of nursing actions. Principles and theories related to sterile technique, for example, have remained constant as equipment and materials changed from reusable supplies to disposable. The nurse who understands the rationale behind sterile technique for various procedures is more able to adapt nursing care to a particular patient using any variety of equipment and supplies available. Principles and theories from disciplines related to nursing, such as anatomy, physiology, microbiology, psychology, and sociology, blend with nursing knowledge and experience to form an integrated base of knowledge that guides the nurse in planning patient care. While the nursing process involves an understanding of the rationale underlying nursing actions, it is not necessary to include this written rationale in documenting the care plan. However, the nursing process is incomplete and potentially unsafe unless nurses base their choices of nursing actions on appropriate rationale. Rationale for nursing actions are included in the various care plans in this text as a teaching tool. In clinical settings, writing rationale for nursing actions consumes much time and space and therefore is inappropriate.

The following example illustrates the principles and theories from various disciplines upon which selection of appropriate nursing actions are based.

NURSING DIAGNOSIS: Sleep pattern disturbance related to hospitalization, pain, and traction as evidenced by inability to fall asleep, reports of fatigue.

NURSING GOAL: Improve nighttime sleep to at least 6 hours/night by 48 hours.

Nursing Interventions	*Rationale*
a. Obtain a sleep history	a. Provides baseline data from which to assess activities that promote or interfere with sleep
b. Assess for factors in the current environment that interfere with sleep and minimize if possible	b. Noise, heat, cold, too hard or soft a bed, roommates, lights, can all interfere with sleep
c. Offer pain medication at HS	c. Pain can interfere with sleep
d. Offer backrub at HS	d. Backrubs help to relax muscles and provide the patient time to talk about any concerns; relaxation and decreased anxiety facilitate sleep
e. Help to reposition in traction	e. Good body alignment decreases strain on muscles and promotes comfort to facilitate sleep
f. Encourage good sleep hygiene 　○ no caffeine after noon meal	○ caffeine is a stimulant

Nursing Interventions	Rationale
○ limit cigarette smoking	○ nicotine can stimulate CNS
○ offer light snack before bed	○ foods high in protein and L-trypto-phan (milk) promote sleep
○ help to follow usual routine for hygiene, time to retire	○ normal habits from home are associated with a good sleeping pattern

Problem-Solving and Selecting Interventions

How does a nurse choose the most appropriate interventions? Some nurses just seem to "know" what to do to help a patient achieve a goal. Others do things because "we have always done it this way." Still others rely on a standard care plan designed for all patients with a similar problem to tell them what to do. Where does a student begin? Nursing students do not base care on intuition. They have to learn how to be effective nurses. That means applying the skills of problem-solving to a particular patient's health problems and the environment in which nursing care is to be given. The following suggestions may be helpful when selecting interventions:

1. Review the nursing diagnosis so the problem and etiology of the problem is clear. For actual problems, try to reduce or eliminate the cause of the problem. If the cause cannot be reduced or eliminated, select interventions to minimize or eliminate the problematic signs and symptoms. For potential problems, select interventions which reduce or eliminate the risk factors. If this is not possible, select interventions to prevent the problem from developing, delay its development, or reduce the severity of the problem when it does develop. For example, insulin dependent diabetics are at risk for tissue damage in the legs and feet. Teaching good foot care and maintenance of blood glucose levels as close to normal as possible may delay or prevent this complication or make it less severe and more easily treated.
2. Examine the goal to have a clear picture of desired outcomes.
3. Consider all possible nursing activities that might help the patient achieve the goal:
   —changes in the environment
   —activities for the patient to perform independently
   —activities to perform with the patient

—activities to perform for the patient
—assistance from other health professionals
—involvement of the patient's friends and family
—changes in the nurse (increased knowledge and skill)

4. Use standard patient care plans as guidelines for developing and
    planning a patient's nursing care. Standard patient care plans may
    be available to you on index cards that will fit in a Kardex care
    plan or in the chart. These standards provide the nurse with gen-
    eral guidelines for patients with particular medical diagnoses, di-
    agnostic studies, or nursing diagnoses. They identify areas for
    assessment, possible patient problems to anticipate, and sug-
    gested outcomes and nursing interventions. They provide the stu-
    dent and the nurse with another resource for planning nursing
    interventions. These standard care plans do not replace the indi-
    vidualized care plan developed by the nurse. Based on the knowl-
    edge about an individual patient, the medical management of health
    problems, the health care setting, and patient and family prefer-
    ences and concerns, the nurse will: fill out the etiology and signs
    and symptoms of the diagnosis, select and individualize goals
    from a list of possible goals, delete inappropriate interventions,
    add new interventions, and individualize general interventions.
    These plans save the nurse time in rewriting common nursing
    interventions but do not replace the process of planning individ-
    ualized care. See Table 3-2.

5. Use the patient and the patient's family as a source of possible
    nursing interventions. Patients may have many good suggestions
    for activities they can perform, with or without nursing assis-
    tance, to achieve a certain goal, based on their past experiences
    and personal preferences. The nurse then uses personal knowl-
    edge and experience to incorporate some of the patient's sugges-
    tions into a plan of care. This collaboration helps to involve pa-
    tients in planning and implementing the type of nursing care they
    receive. By using the patient and family to help plan nursing
    interventions, the nurse considers patient preferences, which usu-
    ally leads to more effective interventions.

6. Use resources, such as nursing fundamentals texts, medical-sur-
    gical nursing texts, and current journal articles. Use the policy
    and procedure manual on the clinical setting for information on
    what is to be done and how to do it in a particular setting.

7. Consider the advantages and disadvantages of possible nursing
    interventions and select those that meet the following criteria:

Table 3–2
Nursing Diagnosis Standard of Care   **Addressograph**

Pain related to _____

("A state in which an individual experiences and reports the presence of severe discomfort or an uncomfortable sensation," NANDA, 1989)
Patient Characteristics: _____

Patient Goals/Outcome Standards:
____ Verbalization that pain has been eliminated or decreased to a level of _____
        on a scale of 1–10 by _____.
                                during _____ .
____ Evaluation: _____
____ Reduction in values of vital signs, P, R, BP, toward normal range
        by _____.
____ Evaluation: _____
Other: _____
____ Evaluation: _____

Nursing Intervention Standards:
    1. Assess pain and related factors.
        a. intensity (1–10) _____
        b. duration _____
        c. character (sharp, dull, shooting, burning) _____
        d. location _____
        e. precipitated by _____

    2. Assess for effectiveness of previous pain relief interventions
        a. previous medication (drug, dose, route, effectiveness on 1–10) ____
            _____
        b. other helpful measures: _____
            _____

    3. Offer _____ (analgesic ordered by MD) q _____ prn.

    4. Encourage use of analgesics before _____
        (pain precipitating activity) at _____ am/pm or _____

    5. Offer relaxation techniques: slow relaxed breathing _____
                                      music _____
                                      backrub _____
                                      heat _____

    6. Assist with repositioning as needed q _____

    7. Encourage use of distracting stimuli: radio, TV, other: _____
        effleurage/skin stroking _____

Developed by _____ date: _____
Evaluated by _____ date: _____
Reviewed/Updated by _____ date: _____

● **Nursing actions must be safe for the patient.** Application of heat to the skin will stimulate circulation, but excessive heat will burn. Nursing actions using heat must ensure that the patient is not burned. Exercising a patient's muscles and joints can be very beneficial; however, if muscles and joints are forced beyond the point of resistance or pain, the nurse can cause injuries.

● **Nursing actions must be congruent with other therapies.** For example, nursing actions must be selected within the safety range ordered by the physician. If the medical order reads "Aspirin (ASA), 2 tablets, q4h, prn," nursing actions cannot plan the administration of aspirin every 2 hours. If the physical therapist is instructing the patient in the use of a walker, the nurse should also use a walker in ambulating the patient.

● **Nursing actions selected are most likely to develop the behavior described in the goal statement.** There may be many different nursing actions that would accomplish the same goal. The nurse attempts to give the patient practice in the specific behavior stated in the goal. For example:

NURSING DIAGNOSIS: Pain related to movement secondary to bone cancer.

NURSING GOAL: Verbalization of pain as less than 3 on a 1–10 scale during hospitalization.

Nursing Actions/Interventions	
May Achieve Goal	*More Likely to Achieve Goal*
a. Offer prescribed pain medication q3–4th prn	a. Assess patient's pain, timing, duration, intensity, and related activities, q3–4h
	b. Administer analgesic ½ hour before physical therapy
	c. Administer analgesic q3h while awake
	d. Assess patient's current methods of dealing with pain and support if possible
	e. Discuss and practice alternate pain relief measures with patient, by March 1 (1) Relaxation

May Achieve Goal	Nursing Actions/Interventions
	More Likely to Achieve Goal
	(2) Alternative sensory stimulation —music —tactile (massage, effleurage, menthol rubs, vibrators) —heat/cold —movies, TV, reading (3) Breathing techniques f. Discuss self-medication for pain, by March 3 g. Discuss effectiveness of pain relief measures with physician and patient h. Encourage use of pain relief measures when discomfort *begins* rather than after it is intense

- **Nursing actions are realistic:**
  —for the patient. Consider age, physical strength, disease, willingness to change behavior, resources.
  —for the number of hospital staff. Will enough people consistently be available to carry out the nursing actions?
  —for the experience and ability of available staff. If most of the staff are unfamiliar with the nursing actions you are suggesting or disagree with it, there is a high probability they will not be carried out.
  —for available equipment. If your nursing actions include the use of any equipment, it should be readily available and the hospital staff should be familiar with its use.
- **Nursing actions consider meeting lower level survival needs before higher level needs.** For example, the following sequence of nursing actions deals with the current need of pain avoidance before asking the patient to deal with potential problems.
  NURSING DIAGNOSIS: Potential for ineffective breathing related to general anesthesia, postop pain.

NURSING GOAL: Normal respiratory rate and lung sounds maintained postop.

NURSING INTERVENTIONS:

a. reduce pain to a level of 4 or less on a 1–10 scale
b. Explain the potential problem and goal to patient.
c. Explain preventive function of the following activities.
    (1) Turning, coughing, and deep breathing at least every 2 hours.
    (2) Early ambulation.
    (3) Use of deep-breathing device, q1 h
d. Explain ways to minimize discomfort during turning and coughing; splinting, analgesics.
e. Offer pain medication 1/2 hour prior to ambulating.
f. Assist patient to:
    (1) TCH q2 h × 24 h
    (2) Ambulate q.i.d. starting first postop day.
    (3) Deep breath ql h while awake × 24 h.
g. Assess lung sounds before and after TCH sessions.

- **Whenever possible, nursing actions should be important to the patient and compatible with personal goals and values.** The patient should understand how the nursing actions will result in achievement of the goal. For example, a man may refuse to do arm and hand exercises because he does not think they are important. If the nursing actions encourage the patient to do activities such as shaving, combing his hair, brushing his teeth, and feeding himself, the arms and hands will still receive the desired exercise. The difference is that the patient values being able to do these self-care activities and can see that they are part of his recovery.

Patient Teaching: An Intervention Strategy

If the nurse assesses a patient and makes a nursing diagnosis with an etiology or risk factors related to a knowledge or performance deficit, a teaching plan will most likely comprise a large portion of the activity in the planning phase of the nursing process. Many plans of care include a teaching component for each goal as the nurse explains what is to be done and why. One of the standards by JCAHO for hospital accreditation states that patient education and patient/family knowledge of self-care are given special consideration in the nursing plan (JCAHO, 1989). Unrealistic fears of a medical procedure and incorrectly taking prescribed medications are examples of problems that could be caused by the patient's belief in erroneous information. Patients with newly diagnosed medical problems are frequently confronted with knowledge deficits concerning the implications of their medical diagnosis and the effect it may have on their life-style. Patients taking on new roles, such as parenting, are frequently concerned about their lack of knowledge and skill in newborn care. Prenatal classes such as Lamaze and CEA will anticipate these learning needs and identify specific areas of newborn care that prospective parents would like to discuss in class. Nursing follow-through in the hospital, after delivery, builds on this information and gives the parents actual practice in caring for their newborn. Similarly, preoperative and postoperative teaching is based on a nursing diagnosis of inadequate knowledge of the surgical experience, complications, and preventive measures. Preoperative teaching is also based on research indicating that an educated patient, knowing what will happen during a procedure, will often experience less pain and anxiety than an unprepared patient. The nursing diagnosis, again, would relate to inadequate or incorrect information about a particular procedure or surgery.

In applying the nursing process to the formulation of a teaching plan, the nurse follows a logical sequence of problem-solving. First, the knowledge deficit is identified based on data obtained during the assessment phase of the nursing process. A goal is then chosen that identifies the learning outcomes. Next, a plan is developed to teach the skill or information to the patient.

For example:

1. NURSING DIAGNOSIS: Knowledge and skill deficit in taking newborn rectal temperature related to first-time parenting.
   [This diagnosis might be written in an alternate form identifying inadequate knowledge and skill as the cause of a potential problem; "Potential for altered health maintenance related to lack of knowledge and skill in newborn temperature assessment."]
   GOAL: Take an accurate rectal temperature on her newborn before discharge, on 3/5.
   NURSING INTERVENTIONS (Teaching Plan):
   1. Discuss when to take baby's temperature; signs and symptoms indicating illness.
   2. Demonstrate how to take rectal temperatures on newborns, 3/4.
   3. Explain safety precautions and when to notify physician for fevers, 3/4.
   4. Provide reinforced practice in taking her newborn's temperature, 3/4.

2. NURSING DIAGNOSIS: Knowledge deficit in taking medications related to forgetting and not reading directions.

[This diagnosis might be written in an alternate form identifying the problem as caused by inadequate knowledge; "Potential for injury related to lack of knowledge of medications and administration."]

GOAL: Demonstrate correct self-administration of medication by 11/3.

NURSING INTERVENTIONS:

1. Check that patient can read all labels on medications, 11/1.
2. Discuss with the patient how to safely take each medication (drug, dose, time, route), 11/1.
3. Provide a clear set of directions in written form regarding medications, 11/1.
4. Supervise patient in hospital with self-administration of prescribed medications, 11/1, 11/2.

When patients learn specific motor skills, the goal selected has a very direct relationship to the diagnosed knowledge or performance deficit. The teaching plan and eventually the evaluation of the patient's ability to perform the skill are usually equally specific. When teaching motor skills, follow the steps of the nursing process:

1. Identify knowledge deficits (NURSING DIAGNOSIS)
   —Inadequate skill in performance of . . .
   —Knowledge deficit in area of . . .
   —Potential for (specify problem) related to lack of knowledge and/or skill in area of . . .
2. Identify the specific behavior the patient will perform based on the diagnosed learning need (GOAL).
3. Teach the specific behavior to the patient (NURSING INTERVENTIONS).
4. Evaluate the patient's ability to perform the specific behavior (EVALUATION).

Evaluating patient learning may be difficult if observable behaviors are not identified as goals during the planning phase. When a patient is developing an understanding of broader concepts or improving cognitive skills, the nurse's teaching plan cannot focus on one specific behavior as evidence of this broader understanding. For example, if the diagnosis relates to inadequate knowledge of infant care, a goal dealing with the isolated behavior of diapering does not provide support for the assumption that the parent is competent in infant care. In this case, the method the nurse may use is the identification of one long-term learning goal and then identification of subsequent several short-term goals that build toward the long-term goal. The long-term goal may be more difficult to state in behavioral terms. The examples of short-term goals should be stated as observable or measurable behaviors. The teaching plan is then directed at the long-term goal by achieving the short-term goals.

Example 1:

NURSING DIAGNOSIS: Knowledge and skill deficit of newborn care related to new parent role.

LONG-TERM GOAL: Parents will safely care for newborn by time of discharge from hospital, on 11/3.

SHORT-TERM GOALS:

1. Demonstrate bathing their newborn, 11/2.
2. Safely take a rectal temperature on newborn, 11/2.
3. Demonstrate cord care for umbilical stump, 11/2.

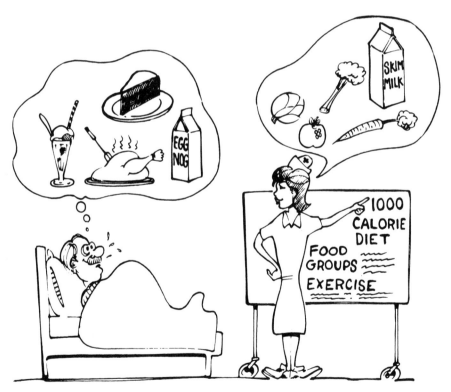

FIGURE 3–4. A good teaching plan does not always guarantee that patient learning will occur.

4. Breast-feeding: 10–15 minutes per breast q2–5 h, by 11/3.
5. Transport newborn home from hospital in infant car seat, 11/3.

TEACHING PLAN: Nursing Interventions

1. Assess readiness for learning infant care (comfort level, fatigue, personal priority needs).
2. Discuss various aspects of infant care: feedings, hygiene, safety, growth and development, behavior.
3. Demonstrate specific infant care skills and provide practice for parents with positive reinforcement.
4. Assist in initiation of breast-feeding and provide specific information on the skill.
5. Provide resources for parents after discharge (people to call when questions or problems arise).

Example 2:

NURSING DIAGNOSIS: Potential for failure in Nursing 101 related to lack of knowledge of the nursing process as evidenced by 2 correct out of 15 points on the unit test.

LONG-TERM GOAL: Student will pass Nursing 101 with a grade of "C" or better by the end of the course.

SHORT-TERM GOALS:

1. Identify five phases of the nursing process, 3/1.
2. Explain nursing diagnosis and how it differs from medical diagnosis, 3/5.
3. Write three nursing diagnoses from a data base, 3/10.
4. Write three nursing goals with observable patient behavior, and criteria of performance, 3/20.
5. Write three sets of nursing interventions to help a patient achieve three different goals by 4/1.
6. Evaluate goal achievement and review care plan by 4/10.

TEACHING PLAN: Nursing Interventions

1. Assess readiness to learn; strengths and interfering factors.
2. Discuss ways to reduce or eliminate factors interfering with learning.
3. Discuss rationale for using the nursing process.
4. Explain, briefly, the relationship between the nursing process patient care, and passing Nsg 101.
5. Assign readings on nursing process.
6. Demonstrate application of nursing process on a hypothetical patient's data base.
7. Use practice exercises for writing nursing diagnoses, goals, and planning actions.

8. Written student assignment: Develop a care plan on four assigned hospital patients showing assessment, diagnosis planning, implementation, and evaluation.

9. Review and critique other students' care plans.

There are several things to consider when developing a teaching plan. Learning is enhanced by using principles of teaching-learning. It is especially important to assess the patient's readiness to learn. An illness, medical problem, or treatment may greatly interfere with learning, particularly in the acute phase of an illness. Medications, fatigue, anxiety, pain, or hunger may all block effective learning. Grief over unexpected, negatively evaluated outcomes related to treatment, medical diagnosis, life-style changes, body changes or prognosis will often delay the desire for learning by the patient. For example, the patient who finally begins to look at her colostomy stump and asks some questions about it, may be ready to listen to some information, while a few days ago she was unwilling to even acknowledge the presence of the colostomy as part of her body. Teaching should be delayed until some of these obstacles have been lessened or eliminated. The nurse also assesses the patient's previous knowledge and skills, building on this prior base. Begin at the level of patient understanding using language understandable to the patient. Individualizing the teaching approach may also lead to improved patient learning. The following principles support these common nursing interventions as part of a teaching plan.

Common Components of a Teaching Plan	Rationale and Scientific Principles
1. Setting a learning goal with the patient.	1. Clarification of desired learning outcomes will guide teaching methods and may serve as a motivating function for the learner.
2. Assessing patient's readiness to learn. a. motivation-recognizes knowledge deficit b. illness/medical problem c. medication/pain d. level of consciousness e. anxiety level f. fatigue	2. A person learns more effectively when the learning experience has personal relevance. A person learns more effectively when a need to learn is perceived. Unmet physical or psychosocial needs such as anxiety, pain, and fatigue have a nega-

Common Components of a Teaching Plan	*Rationale and Scientific Principles*
	tive effect on attention, retention, and ability to learn.
3. Assess patient's current knowledge and motor skill ability. 4. Begin teaching at the patient's current level of understanding or skill performance.	3., 4. Teaching that moves from simple to complex will help to ensure understanding. Simple and complex are relative terms and have meaning only in relationship to the learner's current level of understanding or performance.
5. Provide the patient with an opportunity to practice motor skills after a demonstration. 6. Reinforce patient's efforts to learn whenever possible.	5., 6. An active learner learns and retains more than a passive learner. Practice with feedback and positive reinforcement leads to improved performance and continuance of reinforced behavior.

SUMMARY

During the planning phase of the nursing process, the nurse and the patient set priorities among the identified problems; establish goals showing reduction, prevention; or elimination of the problem; and plan interventions to achieve the goals. A goal is the desired outcome of nursing care in the form of changed patient behavior. For actual nursing diagnoses, the goals indentify patient behavioral outcomes demonstrating a lessening or elimination of the problem. For potential nursing diagnoses, the goals demonstrate the patient maintaining the current level of functioning or prevention of the problem. Goals give direction to nursing actions as do the nursing diagnoses. Long-term goals often demonstrate the maximum level of functioning for the patient or restoration of normal functioning and may take days to months to achieve. Short-term goals describe patient outcome behavior in smaller steps. They might be more appropriate in a critical care setting or when the patient is unstable and the problem must be reduced or eliminated rapidly. Short-term goals may be set in a time frame from hours to days. Progressive short-term goals can be used to show continued progress, in terms of improved level of patient functioning, in the direction of long-term goal achievement. A goal statement contains the patient behavior, the criteria of acceptable performance of that behavior, the time frame

---

A nurse promotes readiness to learn . . .

. . . . . *I was working in the obstetrical unit of a university hospital. A baby had been born a few days ago with a cleft lip and palate. The mother had refused to see or hold the baby since delivery. She stayed in her room, cried frequently and slept off and on during the day. The staff was getting quite fed up with her since the baby was healthy in every other way and she was supposed to take the baby home tomorrow. She had refused the information from the doctor on cleft lip and palate. We had delayed all efforts at teaching infant care based on her refusal to do anything with the baby. She was not ready to learn, but the reality of the hospital setting said she would be discharged with that baby tomorrow, ready or not. The problems of dysfunctional grieving, potential for altered parenting, and even potential for physical harm to the baby were all running through my mind in addition to the knowledge and skill deficit problem. I went in the room and she pulled the covers over her head and said "Go away." "Great start," I thought. "This is going to be a terrific shift!" As I sat down in a chair next to her, I was desperately trying to think of what to do. As honestly as I could, I shared my concerns and frustrations as the nurse for her and her baby. I also wanted her to know I wasn't condemning her or telling her she shouldn't feel the way she felt. "I'm so sorry about your baby, and I know you're very upset. You and the baby are supposed to go home tomorrow and I'm worried because I don't feel like you are ready." I told her what kind of teaching and hands-on care most new mothers are given in the hospital and how they often are still apprehensive about going home. I told her I didn't know how she was feeling or even if she was willing to care for the baby at home. "Your baby is eating very well, acting like all the other babies, crying, sleeping, stooling, and voiding." I was trying to point out what was normal about her baby. After a few moments of silence, I asked the new mother if I could feed her baby in her room because the baby was acting hungry when I left the nursery. The mother agreed, and I held and fed the baby. As I was doing this she reached out and touched the baby's feet and hands and commented on how perfectly they were formed. As I was leaving the room with the baby after the feeding, she asked me to bring her the information on cleft lip and palate that the doctor said he would leave at the nurse's station.*

---

in which the goal should be achieved, and the conditions, if any, under which the behavior will be demonstrated. Goals are realistic, observable, congruent with other health professional's plan of care, and directly related to the nursing diagnosis.

Nursing interventions are those specific activities the nurse plans and implements to help the patient achieve a goal. There are four broad categories of nursing interventions, and the plan of care often incorporates actions from several of these groups: environmental management, physician initiated and ordered interventions, nurse initiated/physician ordered interventions, and nurse initiated/nurse ordered interventions. The last group of interventions is solely within the realm of nursing practice and includes: health teaching, counseling, and referral; specific nursing treatments; assisting with ADLs; assessment of patient status, progress, and response; assistance with problem-solving and providing encouragement and support. Nursing interventions deal with the etiology or risk factor of the problem identified in the nursing diagnosis and try to reduce or eliminate them. If that is not possible, interventions are aimed at lessening the problematic signs and symptoms to assist the patient cope with the problem. Nursing interventions are safe for the patient, specific, congruent with plans of other health professionals, and realistic for the patient, the nurse, and the health care setting.

CASE STUDY: CARE PLAN (Goals, Interventions, and Rationale)

The care plan for Mrs. Witten follows. The data base and nursing diagnoses were developed in Chapters 1 and 2. A standard care plan form is also shown to illustrate how the nursing diagnosis of pain might be individualized.

Care Plan for Mrs. Witten

Nursing Diagnoses	Goals	Interventions	Rationale
Pain secondary to possible cholecystitis	Report of pain at level of 4 or less during hospitalization	1. assess and elim. contributing factors 2. enc. alt. pain mgmt techniques 3. assess q3h; prn analgesic 4. reposition q2h	○ to lessen or elim. cause of pain ○ block or lessen pain perception ○ provide adequate drug level ○ reduce muscle strain ○ good body alignment increases comfort
Fear r/t illness, possible surgery	Patient verbalizes decreased	1. manage pain	○ pain can increase fear

Nursing Diagnoses	Goals	Interventions	Rationale
	fear prior to tests, tx, surgery	2. orient to room, routines	○ decrease fear of unknown
		3. assess knowledge of illness txs, info. from MD	○ begin to teach at pts. level; fear can decrease perception/understanding
		4. explanations; clarify prior to all nsg/medical tests, tx	○ decreases fear of unknown
		5. enc. family support	○ presence of family can decrease fear/ anxiety in pt.
		6. assess for concerns; need to talk	○ verbalizing fears can lessen them and allows nurse to correct misinformation
		7. assess status q1–2h × 12h	○ meets safety need
Alt. health maintenance r/t knowledge deficit on BSE	Patient to demo. BSE before disch.	1. explain impt. of early detection and tx	○ motivational
		2. discuss timing of BSE q mo 1–2 days post menstruation	○ for consistency
		3. teach BSE techniques; normal and abnormal findings	○ for accurate dx of BSE findings
		4. demo/return demo of BSE	○ to assess learning
		5. BSE pamphlet	○ for home reference

Developed by: *L. Atkinson* R.N. date: 6/3/90

89714530
Witten, Laura
6/3/90 room 511
Dr. Ronal/Keller
Addressograph

Nursing Diagnosis Standard Care Plan: Pain

Pain related to *possible cholecystitis 6/3*

("A state in which an individual experiences and reports the presence of severe discomfort or an uncomfortable sensation," NANDA, 1989)
Patient Characteristics: *reports RUQ pain, restless, P96, R28, BP 138/88*

Patient Goals/Outcome Standards:
✓ Verbalization that pain has been eliminated or decreased to a level of *4* on a scale of 1–10 by *1 hr &*
          during *hospitalization* .
___ Evaluation: _____

✓ Reduction in values of vital signs, P, R, BP, toward normal range by *1 hr* .
___ Evaluation: _____
Other: _____
___ Evaluation: _____

Nursing Intervention Standards:
1. Assess pain and related factors.
   a. intensity (1–10) *rated as 8 on admission*
   b. duration *continuous; previously lasted several hours*
   c. character (sharp, dull, shooting, burning) *"acute" sharp*
   d. location *Right Upper quadrant*
   e. precipitated by *unknown*

2. Assess for effectiveness of previous pain relief interventions
   a. previous medication (drug, dose, route, effectiveness on 1–10) ___
     ASA 10gr taken at home "not helpful at all, made me
   b. other helpful measures: *—   nauseated"*

3. Offer *Demerol 50-100mg* (analgesic ordered by MD) q *3-4 h* prn.
           IM

4. Encourage use of analgesics before *tests*
   (pain precipitating activity) at _____ am/pm or _____

5. Offer relaxation techniques: slow relaxed breathing *explained 6/3*
              music *—*
              backrub *q h s*
              heat *—*

6. Assist with repositioning as needed q *4° position of comfort*

7. Encourage use of distracting stimuli: radio, (TV) other: _____
   effleurage/skin stroking *RUQ by patient ad lib*

Developed by *L. Atkinson RN*   date: *6/3/90*
Evaluated by _____ date: _____
Reviewed/Updated by _____ date: _____

CHAPTER 4

Implementation

V. Nursing actions provide for client/patient participation in health promotion, maintenance, and restoration.

VI. Nursing actions assist the client/patient to maximize his health capabilities. (Standards of Nursing Practice, American Nurses' Association, 1973)

Like the other steps comprising the nursing process, the implementation phase consists of several activities: validating the care plan, writing the care plan, giving and documenting nursing care, and continuing to collect data.

Implementation =	Validating Care Plan	+ Documenting Care Plan	+ Giving and Documenting Nursing Care	+ Continuing Data Collection

VALIDATING THE CARE PLAN

When nursing students or inexperienced staff nurses write care plans, it is recommended that they take the proposed care plans to a colleague and request validation. This step does not have to involve a lengthy scheduled consultation but is, rather, a very brief time during which nurses seek the opinion of other nurses. It is important that the student seek appropriate sources for validation. For example, the student may request the clinical instructor or responsible staff nurse to review the care plan. Such qualified sources can evaluate the care plan by using the following questions as guides.

1. Does the plan assure the patient's safety?
2. Is the plan based on sound scientific principles?
3. Is the plan supported by accepted nursing knowledge?
4. Are the nursing diagnoses supported by the data? Are the major defining characteristics present?
5. Do priorities consider patient preferences, physical and psychosocial needs?
6. Do the goals relate to the problems identified in the nursing diagnoses?
7. Do the goals contain a time and patient behavior for evaluation?
8. Can the planned nursing actions realistically assist the patient to achieve the intended goals?
9. Are the nursing actions arranged in a logical sequence?
10. Is the plan individualized to the needs and capabilities of this particular patient?
11. Is the plan congruent with the standards, protocols, and procedures for the particular health care setting? With plans of other health professionals?

Thus, the nurse who provides the validation is reviewing the plan in four major areas:

1. Safety
2. Appropriateness
3. Effectiveness
4. Individualized nursing care

Because of their expertise in nursing care, other nurses are the most frequently used resource for validating. At times, a nurse may wish to utilize another health team member to review some aspect of a nursing care plan. For example, the nurse teaching a diabetic client about a diabetic exchange diet may wish to have a dietitian validate food substitutions requested by the patient.

Occasionally, a nursing student may select an inappropriate person to validate a care plan. Frequently, nursing assistants are very knowledgeable about a specific type of care, having had several years' experience in a particular clinical area. However, the nursing student should not ask nursing assistants to validate a care plan. Nursing assistants may be a source for data in that they may be able to provide information about routines of the clinical area, but they are not planners of nursing care. This is a function of the professional nurse.

Having reviewed the plan with another professional, the student or nurse may wish to share the completed plan with the patient, who is another possible source for validation. The patient can advise the nurse if any aspect of the plan is unacceptable. This gives patients another opportunity to participate in planning their own care. In summary, to validate the plan is to request another appropriate professional and the patient, if possible, to give the plan approval for implementation.

DOCUMENTING THE NURSING CARE PLAN

To retain a nursing care plan for the exclusive use of one nurse is to defeat a primary purpose of care plans. In order to get the maximum effect, a care plan must get the maximum press!

A nurse may plan a patient care conference as a "press conference" for a completed care plan. At such a meeting the nurse summarizes data, problems, goals, and planned actions. The nurse spends most of the time focusing on presenting the care plan to other nurses. At such a time the nurse may also gain new information to add to the care plan. This conference may be used as a problem-solving session during which a nurse may request assistance from colleagues to further develop a care plan.

Interdisciplinary care conferences involve various professionals such as the physician, physical therapist, social worker, dietician, and chaplain in addition to the patient's primary nurse. All these professionals work together to develop a plan of care for the patient, especially focusing on long-term goals and interventions. The patient and family participate in this problem-solving group whenever possible.

The change of shift report is another time when the nurse shares concerns about patients, seeks additional data or suggestions from colleagues, identifies problems, sets priorities, identifies goals, and plans interventions. This process will direct the nurse's activities during the coming 8 hour shift. The nurse can delegate or clarify activities for other health team members so everyone knows what is important to assess and report and what to do for or with the patient/family over the next few hours.

Another communication tool following the sequence of activities in the nursing process is a charting format known as a problem oriented medical record (POMR). The plan of care in such a system then takes the form of SOAP or (SOAPIER) notes. The word SOAP is used as an acronym for

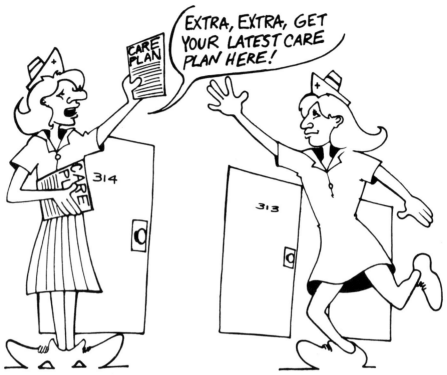

FIGURE 4-1.   A nursing care plan must be shared, in order to be effective.

subjective data, objective data, assessment, and plan. Some formats add the use of the letters IER to include implementation, evaluation, and reassessment.

Another popular format is "focus charting." The focus is often the diagnostic category or an identified nursing diagnosis. The charting then involves continued reporting of data on the problem, an interpretation of that data in relationship to the problem, changes or additions to nursing actions, and evaluation of outcomes after implementing these interventions.

Other hospitals use a nursing Kardex as a system of organizing care plans. A nursing Kardex is a file that contains the nursing care plans. Each plan is recorded on an oversized index card or large folded sheet of paper. Kardex forms may include space for medical treatments, diagnostic procedures, and other schedules. Still other institutions have adopted 8 1/2 inch × 11 inch nursing care plan forms, which have the advantage of corresponding to standard chart size.

Some computerized hospitals are using the computer to generate a standardized care plan for a patient with a specific diagnosis. The nurse begins with this care plan and then modifies it to meet the needs of the individual patient. Other heath care settings are "filling in the blanks" to individualize a pre-printed standard care plan developed by more expert nurses.

The form of the written care plan may vary from institution to institution, but it should be a useful tool for communicating. Most Kardexes will include space for nursing diagnoses, goals, nursing orders, and evaluation in an abbreviated form. A written care plan may be condensed but must convey all essential information. Often nurses will use worksheets to record those problems, goals, and interventions that will probably be accomplished during their 8-hour shift.

This 8-hour plan does not need to be written as a permanent care plan, although the nursing care must be documented in the patient's chart and a report given to the following shift of nurses. The written care plan should be used to communicate goals that cover several shifts or more and require the coordinated efforts of several nurses over a period of time.

The following suggestions will assist the nurse to write a care plan on a Kardex or any similar form.

1. Abbreviate whenever possible, using standardized medical or English symbols.
2. Choose key words to communicate ideas; do not write whole sentences.
3. Refer people to procedure books rather than trying to include all the steps for a procedure on a written plan.
4. Category headings should include nursing diagnoses, goals, nursing actions, and evaluations.
5. The nursing diagnosis with the related goal and nursing actions should appear next to each other on the care plan.
6. Include a date for evaluation of each goal.
7. All long-term goals should be written. Nursing actions directly related to long-term goals should also be written. If a short-term goal will be evaluated within the nurse's 8-hour shift, it is not necessary to include it on the written form. It is necessary to document the nursing care.
8. Short-term goals that cannot be met within an 8-hour shift should be written in order that other nurses can continue the plan of care.
9. Long-term goals being met by a series of short-term goals have both the long-term goals and the progressive short-term goals on

the Kardex. The accompanying actions for short-term goals are included. If the short-term goal is to be met during the next few hours by the nurse writing the care plan, the nurse should write the next progressive short-term goal and nursing actions.

   10.   When goals are evaluated, they should be signed and dated by the responsible nurse.

   11.   All nursing interventions (actions, orders, or whatever term is being used) should be signed by the registered nurse responsible for writing them.

   The nursing care plan for Mrs. Witten as it might appear on a Kardex is at the end of this chapter.

GIVING AND DOCUMENTING NURSING CARE

At last! The nurse now has a plan that will individualize the care given to a patient. Now the nurse is ready to give the care as planned. Even though the nurse has developed an excellent care plan, occasionally (and in the hospital it seems to be the rule), situations occur that interfere with implementing the plan. The patient may be scheduled for emergency surgery. A patient may be in great pain, which alters priorities. Visitors may arrive and the patient is eager to spend time with them. In each case the nurse may be unable to implement the care plan without making some modifications. There are times when the nurse believes that performance of certain assessments, treatments, and activities are necessary for the patient's physical safety. Patients, family, and other health care workers may then have to reset their priorities, reschedule or modify what they were planning. For example, a newborn with an admitting rectal temperature of 96°F is hypothermic and interventions to stabilize and raise the temperature should be implemented immediately. Any activities with the newborn, such as bathing or removing the baby from the warmer, might worsen the problem or interfere with treatment and should be delayed until the temperature is back in the normal range. The nurse discusses the problem, goal, and interventions with the family and others working with this newborn. The nurse may problem-solve with the family at this time to identify alternate ways to meet family needs while still guaranteeing treatment for the hypothermia. For example, parents could keep the baby in their room under the warmer for picture taking and to prevent separation.

   Finally, as a last step in implementation, the nurse documents the care given to patients. The nurse is guided by the old maxim "If it is not recorded, it has not been done." If evidence of implementation does not exist in the patient's permanent record, it would seem that the plan has not

---

Even the best laid plans sometimes run amok . . .

. . . . . *I was a nursing instructor working with a young attractive, single male nursing student on the labor and delivery area. We had discussed how uncomfortable he felt and he jokingly said his goal for this clinical rotation was to avoid seeing a birth. We laughed but I said I could accept that as long as he was responsible for the theoretical content and had some experience with the monitors and assessments. His eyes lit up as he scanned the Kardex and chose to follow two women in preterm labor where the goal of medical management was to stop their labor. When he began to follow them, both women were experiencing almost no contractions but had on fetal and uterine monitors. He was feeling quite smug with his assignment and relieved that it looked like his personal goal was a "given." As he walked past a patient's room on the way to the desk, he heard the patient scream out "Help! Help! The baby's coming!" He confided later the thought crossed his mind to keep on walking but he stopped and went in. The woman was in a small panic and a look under the covers at the bulging perineum confirmed the reason for her distress. Just then the staff nurse the student was working with on the cases in preterm labor came into the room responding to the call light. "Saved!" he thought as he headed for the door. His nurse told him, in no uncertain terms, he was helping her and within a few minutes they had delivered the baby. I knew nothing of all this but I ran into him about 15 minutes after the birth and casually asked if he had gotten down for supper yet. "Supper!" he replied. "I just delivered a baby! I may never eat again!"*

---

been followed and the efforts of the nurse have been wasted. In addition, following the nursing interventions planned by a colleague is a way that nurses support each other in developing accountability for nursing care. Few nurses would omit giving or documenting a medication ordered by a physician. The implementation of nursing interventions is equally important to the well-being of patients and thus deserves to be treated seriously, respectfully, and with full accountability.

CONTINUING DATA COLLECTION

Throughout the process of implementation the nurse continues to collect data. As the patient's condition changes, the data base changes, subsequently requiring revising and updating of the care plan. Data gathered while giving nursing care may also be used as evidence for evaluation of goal achievement, which will be discussed in the next chapter.

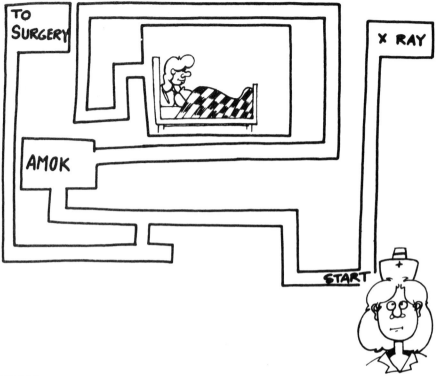

FIGURE 4–2.   Even the best laid plans sometimes run amok.

SUMMARY

Implementation is the fourth step in the nursing process and the focus is on the nurse working with the patient to carry out the plan of care. Implementation consists of validating the care plan (is it a safe, reasonable plan indicating quality nursing care?), documenting and communicating it, but the primary component is actually giving care to the patient. The nurse then documents this care and the patient's response to it in the chart. As the nurse gives care, assessment of the patient continues. This is done not only to see how the patient responds to the nursing interventions but to provide increased information for revising the plan of care as patient status changes. The patient is an active participant in care, working with the nurse to adapt interventions as they are given and having the right to refuse or request interventions. The nurse is flexible, open to suggestions and changing patient priorities but committed to helping the patient understand and accept nursing care to promote health and reduce, eliminate, or prevent problems.

CASE STUDY: ABBREVIATED CARE PLAN

Abbreviated Care Plan for Mrs. Witten

Nursing Diagnoses	Goals	Interventions	Evaluation
Pain secondary to possible cholecystitis	Report of pain at level of 4 or less during hospitalization	1. assess and elim. contributing factors 2. enc. alt. pain mgmt techniques 3. assess q3h; prn analgesic 4. reposition q2h	_____
Fear r/t illness, possible surgery	Patient verbalizes decreased fear prior to tests, tx, surgery	1. manage pain 2. orient to room, routines 3. assess knowledge of illness txs, info. from MD 4. explanations; clarify prior to all nsg/medical tests, tx 5. enc. family support 6. assess for concerns; need to talk 7. assess status q1–2h x 12h	_____
Alt. health maintenance r/t knowledge deficit on BSE	Patient to demo. BSE before disch.	1. explain impt of early detection and tx 2. discuss timing of BSE q mo 1–2 days post menstruation 3. teach BSE techniques; normal and abnormal findings 4. demo/return demo of BSE 5. BSE pamphlet	_____

Developed by: *L. atkinson RN*   date: 6/3/90

CHAPTER 5

Evaluation

VII. The client's/patient's progress or lack of progress toward goal achievement is determined by the client/patient and the nurse.

VIII. The client's/patient's progress or lack of progress toward goal achievement directs reassessment, reordering of priorities, new goal setting, and revision of the plan of nursing care. (Standards of Nursing Practice, American Nurses' Association, 1973)

Evaluation is the last chapter and the final step in the nursing process, yet like the other steps, it is an ongoing activity. There are two parts to evaluation: evaluation of goal achievement and review of the nursing care plan.

$$\text{Evaluation} = \frac{\text{Evaluation of}}{\text{Goal Achievement}} + \frac{\text{Review of the}}{\text{Nursing Care Plan}}$$

EVALUATION OF GOAL ACHIEVEMENT

The purpose of the first part of evaluation is to decide whether the patient has achieved the goal selected during the planning phase of the nursing process. The goal is evaluated at the time or date specified in the goal statement. While giving patient care, the nurse is continuously collecting new data about the patient. Some of this information will be used for evaluation of goal achievement. When evaluating goal achievement, the nurse returns to the goal statement in the care plan. What was the specific patient behavior stated in the goal? Was the patient able to perform the behavior by the time allowed in the goal statement? Was the patient able to perform the behavior as well as described in the criteria part of the goal statement? The answers to these questions are the basis for an evaluation of goal achievement.

The only thing that is evaluated is the patient's ability to demonstrate the behavior described in the goal statement. Nursing actions are not evaluated at this point and are not part of the evaluation statement. Effectiveness of the nursing actions and teaching plans will be examined during review of the overall plan of care. The nurse may have given the world's fastest bedbath, but that is not important for evaluating goal achievement. If the goal was to have the patient relax and sleep for several hours, the nurse evaluates the patient's behavior. Did the patient sleep for several hours? The skill with which a nurse performs various procedures is important and will affect goal achievement. However, when an evaluative statement is written, it is the patient's behavior that is assessed. *The outcome of nursing care in the form of changed patient behavior is the focus of goal evaluation.*

Writing an Evaluative Statement

There are two parts to an evaluative statement: a decision on how well the goal was achieved, and the patient data or behavior that supports this decision. The nurse has three alternatives when deciding how well a goal was met: (1) goal met, (2) goal partially met, and (3) goal not met.

If the patient was able to demonstrate the behavior by the specific time or date in the goal statement, the goal was met. If the patient was able to demonstrate the behavior but not as well as the nurse had specified in the goal statement, the goal was partially met. If the patient was unable or unwilling to perform the behavior at all, the goal was not met.

$$\text{Evaluative Statement} = \begin{matrix} \text{Goal Met} \\ \text{Goal Partially Met} \\ \text{Goal Not Met} \end{matrix} + \begin{matrix} \text{Actual Patient Be-} \\ \text{havior as Evidence} \end{matrix}$$

In the evaluative statement, the nurse includes a description of the patient's actual behavior as the individual tries to demonstrate the behavior identified in the goal. For example, if the behavior identified in the goal was for the patient to report some degree of pain relief, the nurse talks with the patient regarding severity of pain, following the nursing interventions to help relieve it. The patient's response about the severity of current pain makes up the second part of the evaluative statement. Another example might be:

1. Nursing Diagnosis: Activity intolerance related to prolonged bedrest.
    Goal Statement: Patient will walk length of hall and back by 2/7.
    Goal Evaluation (done on 2/7 or earlier):
    Goal achieved; patient walked length of hall and back.
    Goal partially achieved; patient walked length of hall but too tired to walk back.
    Goal not achieved; patient refused to walk.
    Goal not achieved; patient unable to bear his own weight.

2. Nursing Diagnosis: Impaired tissue integrity related to pressure and poor circulation.
    Goal Statement: 2/7 Decubitus ulcer (bedsore) will be healed in 1 month.
    Goal Evaluation (done on 3/7 or earlier):
    Goal met; decubitus ulcer healed.

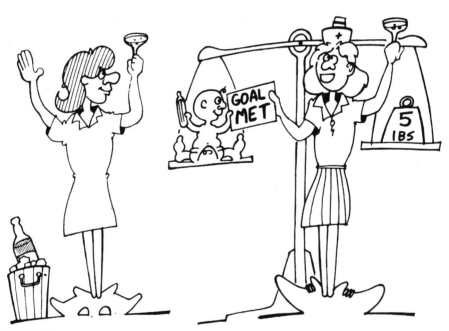

FIGURE 5–1.   Goal met—congratulations! Preterm newborn reached 5 lb goal weight by 10/12.

Goal partially met; decubitus ulcer still present but is 1/2 the size and dry.

Goal not met; decubitus ulcer broken open and draining.

3. Nursing Diagnosis: Noncompliance with assigned reading in *Understanding the Nursing Process* related to belief content is "boring."

Goal Statement: After finishing Chapter 5, the student will state this nursing process book is the most interesting book ever read.

Goal Evaluation (done when the student finishes Chapter 5):

Goal met; student stated this book was the most interesting book ever read and asked for an "A" in the course.

Goal partially met; student said this book was about as interesting as any other course books, and asked for a "C" in the course.

Goal not met; student lost book and asked for a class withdrawal slip.

Patient Participation and Evaluation

Evaluation of goal achievement is done with the patient whenever possible. It may also be done with the patient's family. It is not just the nurse's assessment of the patient's ability to achieve a goal that is important. The patient's perception is also important since the problem identified in the nursing diagnosis is the patient's problem and not the nurse's. The patient who evaluates personal goal achievement is a partner with the nurse and receives feedback on progress toward eliminating or reducing the original problem identified in the nursing diagnosis. When a patient successfully achieves a goal mutually set with the nurse, that person receives positive reinforcement to continue efforts toward a higher level of functioning.

When evaluating goal achievement, the nurse is responsible for documenting both parts of the goal statement. The nurse doing the evaluation with the patient includes the date the evaluation was done, whether or not the goal was achieved, subjective and objective data related to the patient's behavior compared to the behavior identified in the goal, and the nurse's signature. This information is all recorded on the care plan. See Table 5-1. The care plan for Mrs. Witten, developed in Chapters 1, 2, and 3 is presented in Table 5-2 with the addition of evaluation of goal achievement.

Table 5–1   Goal Evaluation

Nursing Diagnoses	Goals	Evaluation
1. Knowledge deficit of diabetic management related to new diagnosis	1. Maintains control of blood glucose levels between 80–180 m/dl (long-term goal)	
	a. accurately checks blood glucose level QID before discharge (short-term goal)	a. goal met; correctly performed self blood glucose checks x 4 *L. Atkinson RN 11/11*
	b. lists signs and symptoms of hyperglycemia and hypoglycemia by 11/12 (short-term goal)	b. goal partly met; lists S&S for hypoglycemia, confused on hyperglycemia *L. Atkinson RN 11/12*
	c. states actions to take for hyper/hypoglycemia by 11/12 (short-term goal)	c. goal met; stated corrective actions for hyper/hypoglycemia *L. Atkinson RN 11/12*
	d. correctly administers own insulin by discharge (short-term goal)	d. goal met; correctly gave self mixed dose of NPH and regular insulin x 2 days *L. Atkinson RN 11/14*
	e. correctly explains how to adjust diet and insulin with short-term illness by 11/13 (short-term goal)	e. goal not met; states never sick and does not think adjustment necessary *L. Atkinson RN 11/13*
2. Fear related to development of diabetes and complications which may develop	2. Patient to state decreased fear and confidence in ability to reduce risks of complications by 12/14 (long-term goal)	2. Goal met. States "it will be a constant worry but I am not as terrified as I was. Lots of people do fine managing their diabetes". *L. Atkinson RN 12/14*
3. Body image disturbance related to diagnosis of insulin dependent diab. as evidenced by anger over need to take insulin and change life-style	3. Verbalizations of acceptance of diab. and willingness to make changes by 12/14 (long-term goal)	3. Goal not met; patient states anger about dx and states it's not fair. "I just hate taking shots; it makes me feel like a drug addict." *L. Atkinson RN 12/14*

CASE STUDY: GOAL EVALUATION

**Table 5–2 Abbreviated Care Plan for Mrs. Witten
(Evaluation Added)**

Nursing Diagnoses	Goals	Interventions	Evaluation
Pain secondary to possible cholecystitis	Report of pain at level of 4 or less during hospitalization	1. assess and elim. contributing factors 2. enc. alt. pain mgmt techniques 3. assess q3h; prn analgesic 4. reposition q2h	Goal partially met; pt. reported pain tolerable with analgesic but still hurts. 6/6/90 *L. atkinson* RN
Fear r/t illness, possible surgery	Patient verbalizes decreased fear prior to tests, tx, surgery	1. manage pain 2. orient to room, routines 3. assess knowledge of illness txs, info. from MD 4. explanations; clarify prior to all nsg/medical tests, tx 5. enc. family support 6. assess for concerns; need to talk 7. assess status q1–2h x 12h	Goal partly met; reporting "scared" but better than at admission. 6/5/90 *L. atkinson* RN
Alt. health maintenance r/t knowledge deficit on BSE	Patient to demo. BSE before disch.	1. explain impt of early detection & tx 2. discuss timing of BSE q mo 1–2 days post menstruation 3. teach BSE techniques; normal & abnormal findings 4. demo/return demo of BSE 5. BSE pamphlet	Goal met; pt demo. BSE correctly 6/8/90 *M. Burns* R.N.

Developed by: *L. atkinson* RN   date: 6/3/90

REVIEW OF THE NURSING CARE PLAN

Following evaluation of goal achievement, the nurse repeats the activities in the nursing process by reviewing the plan of care. This is done whether the goal was achieved or not. Review of the nursing care plan keeps the plan current and responsive to the patient's changing needs. The process of nursing is not just sequential, consisting of steps 1 through 5 and then you are done. The process of nursing is cyclical in nature with the steps of assessment, diagnosis, planning, implementation, and evaluation viewed as a circle with one step leading to another. The nursing care a person receives reflects the changing health status of the patient, medical treatment changes, environmental changes, and the changing needs of the patient and family.

$$
\begin{array}{l}
\text{Review of} \\
\text{the Nursing} \\
\text{Care Plan}
\end{array}
=
\text{Reassessment} +
\begin{array}{l}
\text{Review of} \\
\text{Nursing} \\
\text{Diagnoses}
\end{array}
+ \text{Replanning} +
\begin{array}{l}
\text{Review of} \\
\text{Implementation}
\end{array}
$$

Review of the care plan using the nursing process consists of activities already described in the previous chapters: reassessment, review of diagnoses, replanning, and review of implementation. This process of review results in an updated plan for nursing care, which is then implemented and evaluated, leading again to review as part of evaluation.

Reassessment

The process of reassessment results in an updated information base on the patient. The nurse is continually assessing the patient during all interactions. This accumulation of new data will now supplement the original data base from which the care plan was developed. After evaluation of goal achievement, the nurse looks at the data, the diagnosis, goals, and interventions again. In reassessment, the nurse:

1. Examines original data (related to the problem and goal just evaluated) to decide whether it still accurately represents the patient's status.
2. Examines new data gathered during interventions with the client to: clarify the original problem, its etiology, and related signs and symptoms; serve as a data base for a new nursing diagnosis.

Review of Nursing Diagnoses

The outcome of reviewing the nursing diagnoses is a care plan containing only those diagnoses that are current or potential problems for the patient. This may result in the same diagnoses continuing as part of the plan, new diagnoses being added, and resolved diagnoses eliminated. During the process of reviewing diagnoses, the nurse:

1. Analyzes new data to determine if a new or potential problem exists and makes a new nursing diagnosis as needed. This addition is then documented in the care plan.
2. Analyzes original and new data including data from goal evaluation to determine if original diagnoses are still accurate, current problems requiring nursing care. If they are still accurate and current, these diagnoses remain on the care plan as originally written.
3. Clarifies diagnostic statements to reflect any changes or additions in etiology or signs and symptoms discovered during ongoing assessment with the patient. These changes are then added to the original diagnostic statement in the chart.
4. Analyzes original and new data, and data from goal evaluation to determine if the problem has been resolved and no longer requires nursing care. "Diagnosis resolved" is then documented and dated on the chart and nurses no longer perform the interventions associated with that diagnosis.

If the goal was not achieved, reassessment and review of the diagnoses may help to point out reasons for this, such as inaccurate or incomplete data, inaccurate analysis of the data resulting in an invalid nursing diagnosis, or the development of new problems that interfered with the original plan. If the goal was met and the problem resolved, the nurse considers the need for preventive nursing care if the patient is still at risk.

Replanning

The outcome of this activity will be a plan of care ready for implementation based on current problems, with goals and interventions adjusted to best reflect the patient's abilities and preferences. Ineffective interventions can be eliminated, effective ones emphasized, and new approaches included to facilitate movement toward goal achievement. During this step, the nurse:

1. Reexamines priorities among the diagnoses and determines if they are still appropriate. Priorities are reordered as needed based on new data, new diagnoses, medical management, and expected date for discharge, transfer, surgery, and so on.

2. Examines previous goals and determines if they are still appropriate outcome behaviors or if the patient's status has changed making the goals unrealistic. The behavior, time frame, criteria,

---

A student in nursing discovers the problem when review of the care plan is not complete . . .

. . . *I was teaching with a group of 3rd quarter freshman nursing students on an orthopedic clinical area. We had spent a lot of classroom and clinical time on developing nursing care plans but in the actual clinical setting the students found standard care plans being used. Nurses would diagnose a problem area based on patient assessment and then use the NANDA approved diagnoses with suggested goals and interventions all typed out. The nurse was to individualize this care plan based on knowledge of the patient and the medical treatment plan and put it in the chart. Well, the students were thrilled. This was a lot better than creating a care plan from scratch. A few words and marks on a pre-printed form and they were done. One student in particular was irritated with the nursing faculty for making the students do all this work of care planning when in reality the nurses in the hospital were using care plan forms developed by experienced nurses from the health care facility. The Kardex only contained a list of partially written diagnoses such as "Pain" or "Impaired Physical Mobility." I expressed my concern that care plan review could easily be neglected by such a process because many nurses do not use the chart as a guide to nursing care but continue to use the Kardex which no longer contains the plan of care. My fears were dismissed as unrealistic because on the flow sheet in the patient's chart each shift documented, by initialing, that the care plan had been reviewed. About an hour later, that student called me over and said she had a real problem. The patient she had been caring for all shift was a four day postop amputee. The student had found the plan of care and knew she had to read it because I would be around asking if it was updated. The diagnosis of "Pain related to poor circulation and skin breakdown areas on left lower leg" was still in the chart as originally individualized by the admitting nurse over a week ago. That lower leg had been amputated four days ago. "How could this happen?" she asked. I just smiled. The students had a great postconference discussion on charting, care planning, legal documentation, and ethics.*

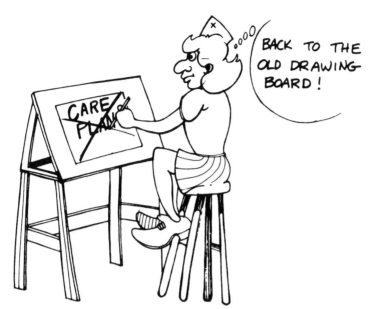

FIGURE 5–2. Review of the nursing care plans leads to revision reflecting the most current status of the patient.

and condition can all be altered to make the goal more appropriate and achievable, while still moving toward problem resolution.

3. Identifies new goals for new diagnoses and selects interventions. These then are documented in the chart.

4. Examines nursing interventions selected in the original plan and determines whether they should continue unchanged or whether a different approach would be more effective. Any changes, additions, or deletions are then documented in the chart as part of the updated care plan.

The following example illustrates review of the plan of care. The reader should understand these steps are not written out as such in the plan as are diagnoses, goals, and interventions but the plan of care is continually updated using whatever form of documentation the health care setting has implemented. Therefore the nurse will not find the headings of "reassessment," "review of diagnoses," "review of plan," or "review of implementation" as part of the care plan. These steps indicate the *process* the nurse goes through to reach the *product* of an effective, current plan of care.

Nursing Diagnoses	Goals	Interventions	Evaluation
Potential for impaired tissue integrity r/t cast on left leg. 6/4/90	Tissue to remain intact, with normal sensation while hospitalized in cast	1. Assess CMS qh x 24 then q4h 2. Elevate leg in good alignment x 24h 3. Turn and reposition q2h until cast dry 4. Pad friction areas at knee and toes	Date: 6/6/90 Eval: Goal met; tissue intact at discharge

Developed by: *L. atkinson* R.N. 6/4/90

Signature:
of nurse evaluating
L. atkinson R.N.

New Data	New Updated Goal	New Interventions
1. 6/6 discharge to home in cast. 2. Skin intact at discharge. (Original Dx still appropriate)	Tissue to remain intact, with normal sensation while casted	1. Assess knowledge of S&S of inadeq circ., pressure, friction 2. Teach home care of cast 3. Enc. elevation when sitting at home/work

Developed by: *L. atkinson* 6/6/90

Review of Implementation

During review of implementation, the nurse examines what actually happened with the patient during nursing care. Factors such as the environment, the nurse's skills and knowledge, and the patient's responses are considered. This is where the nurse evaluates personal behavior in relation to giving patient care. Does the nurse require further skills or information to be more effective? Did the nurse's personal feelings affect the quality of care delivered to the patient? Were the interventions realistic in terms of time and resources? Were the interventions carried out by other nursing personnel? If not, why not? Were the interventions too vague or misinterpreted? Review of what occurred during implementation of the original nursing plan of care may point out problems that can be corrected as the plan is updated. This is especially important when the goal was not achieved. Evaluation, consisting of evaluation of goal achievement and review of the nursing plan of care, helps the nurse develop the skills of writing realistic and effective care plans for dealing with patient's problems.

Without reassessment by a nurse the patient's recovery may have been at risk . . .

. . . . *I hate to float to another area when our floor isn't busy. But float me they did. I usually worked on the burn unit and really felt competent working with the patients but they floated me to an oncology/chemotherapy unit. Different treatments, different problems, different things to assess, lots of drugs to look up. One of my patients was a man admitted to the hospital for workup of an unidentified blood disorder that had been causing him trouble for 15 years. The focus of care was on his hematologic problem, pain management, and possible narcotic addiction. On the Kardex it was noted that he had a partial thickness burn on the palm of his hand that had been treated in the emergency room. The last date on the treatment order for the burn was a week ago. I knew what a burn of that degree should look like if it was healing properly but his hand didn't look the way it should. I assessed the hand and reviewed the ordered treatment based on my own knowledge of burn healing, complications, and available treatments. I discussed my concerns with the head nurse who admitted being unfamiliar with burn therapy and complications. She then notified the responsible physician who then asked for a consult from one of the physicians on the burn unit. The doctor came down and reassessed the burn and the treatment and told me it was a good thing I had questioned the healing and treatment. He said I had probably saved the patient from an infection and possible sepsis by my assessment and action. I guess some days nurses are meant to float.*

SUMMARY

Evaluation is the final step in the nursing process. The first part of evaluation involves evaluation of goal achievement. To do this, the nurse returns to the goal statement to review the outcome behavior identified which would indicate a lessening or elimination of an actual patient problem. Using the new data collected during implementation of the care plan, the nurse evaluates the patient's ability to demonstrate the goal behavior. A range of outcomes can be expected from complete ability to demonstrate the behavior as stated in the goal to complete inability or unwillingness to demonstrate the behavior. This goal evaluation is documented in the chart with a description of the patient's outcome behavior as evidence of the degree of goal achievement.

The second part of evaluation is to review the plan of care. This involves updating the data base, deciding if original diagnoses are still accurate, adding new diagnoses or identifying original ones as resolved, revising the goals and interventions based on more complete information on the patient and the effectiveness of the original plan, and finally implementing the updated plan. This is again followed by goal evaluation and care plan review to reflect the dynamic state of the patient. (See Figure 5-3.)

FIGURE 5–3. Evaluation flow chart.

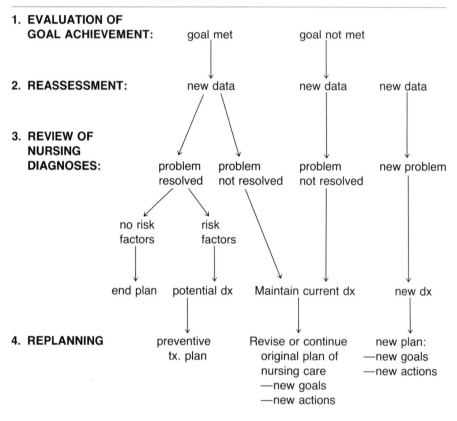

5. REVIEW OF IMPLEMENTATION: How could the nurse do or schedule things differently to be more effective? Improved skill or knowledge base needed? Alter priorities? Better assessments? Help from other health care professionals? Better delegation of responsibility to other nursing staff?

CASE STUDY: REVIEW OF CARE PLAN

The care plan of Mrs. Witten follows with the addition of the second part of evaluation, review of the plan of care. The updated abbreviated care plan demonstrates how it might appear on a nursing Kardex or in the chart. Goal evaluation on a standard care plan form for the diagnostic category of "Pain" as it might be individualized for Mrs. Witten is also shown.

Abbreviated Care Plan for Mrs. Witten (Updated Postop)

Revisions in the care plan are indicated with a * to make changes more obvious but would not appear this way on an actual plan of care.

Reassessment: new data 6/6/90
—transferred back to station 3 hours postop, cholecystectomy
—IV infusing at 125cc/h, D5LR 1000cc to run x 3 liters
—Penrose drain in place draining blood-tinged bile
—½ inch diameter drainage area on incisional dressing
—nasogastric tube in place draining gastric contents on low suction
—NPO day of surgery, then clear liquids as tol. first postop day
—shallow respirations; 22–24 breaths/min
—patient reports severe incisional pain with movement, deep breathing
—refuses to cough; "hurts too much"
—moist breath sounds in lower left lung
—patient states, "I'm so glad it is over! What a relief"
—pulse 92, BP 142/70
—Demerol 50–100mg IM, prn pain
—Tylenol #3 1–2 tabs prn pain, first postop day

Nursing Diagnoses	Goals	Interventions	Evaluation
Pain secondary to possible cholecystitis 6/3/90	Report of pain at level of 4 or less during hospitalization	1. assess and elim. contributing factors 2. enc. alt. pain mgmt techniques 3. assess q3h prn analgesic 4. reposition q2h	Goal partially met; pt. reported pain tolerable with analgesics but still hurts. 6/6/90 *L. Atkinson* R.N.
*Pain related to surgery 6/6/90	*Report of pain at level of 4 or less with use of analgesics during hospitalization	*1. explain analgesia options: type and dose based on pain *2. enc. use of anal. before pain severe	

Nursing Diagnoses	Goals	Interventions	Evaluation
		*3. pain assessment q 3–4h	
		*4. assist with repositioning q2h	
		*5. demo splinting incision for movement/ coughing/deep breath	
		*6. call light in reach	
		*7. backrub at hs	
Fear r/t illness, possible surgery 6/3/90	Patient verbalizes decreased fear prior to tests, tx, surgery	1. manage pain as above 2. orient to room, routines 3. assess knowledge of illness txs, info. from MD 4. explanations; clarify prior to all nsg/medical tests, tx 5. enc. family support 6. assess for concerns/need to talk 7. assess status q1–2h x 12h	Goal partly met; reporting "scared" but better than at admission. 6/5/90 *L. Atkinson RN* *Goal met; problem resolved. Pt expresses relief surgery over 6/6
Alt. health maintenance r/t knowledge deficit on BSE 6/3/90	Patient to demo. BSE before disch.	*Schedule teaching for 6/8 1. explain impt of early detection and tx 2. discuss timing of BSE q mo 1–2 days post menstruation 3. teach BSE techniques; normal and abnormal findings 4. demo/return demo of BSE 5. BSE pamphlet	

Nursing Diagnoses	Goals	Interventions	Evaluation
*Ineffective air-way clearance re-lated to pain as evidenced by shal-low resp. at 24, refusal to cough or deep breathe, moist breath sounds in L lower lung. 6/6/90	*Clear breath sounds by 6/7.	*1. explain need to cough deep breathe *2. assess breath sounds q4h *3. SMI x 3 qh (sus-tained maximal inspiration held for several sec-onds before ex-hale) *4. inspirometer q2h x 48h *5. reposition q2h *6. enc. use of anal-gesics, splinting to decrease pain so pt will cough; enc coughing q2h until lungs clear *7. begin ambulation 1st postop day and advance as tol.	

Developed by: *L. atkinson* RN   **date:** 6/3/90

Reviewed/updated: M.E. Murray RN   **date:** 6/6/90

Nursing Diagnosis Standard Care Plan: Pain

Pain related to *possible cholecystitis 6/3*
6/6 Pain related to surgery for cholecystitis
("A state in which an individual experiences and reports the presence of severe
discomfort or an uncomfortable sensation," NANDA, 1989)
Patient Characteristics: *reports RUQ pain, restless; P96, R28, BP 138/88*
6/6 Pt. reports post-op pain as 6, continuous, dull, P90 R20,
Patient Goals/Outcome Standards: *BP 130/74*
✓ Verbalization that pain has been eliminated or decreased to a level of __4__
on a scale of 1–10 by __1 hr &__
during *hospitalization*
6/3 Evaluation: *Goal partly met; pt. reports pain tolerable*
c̄ analgesics but still hurts.
✓ Reduction in values of vital signs, P, R, BP, toward normal range
by __1 hr__.
6/3 Evaluation: *Goal partially met; p88, R20, BP 130/76*
Other: *6/6 Pt. to state pain maintained at 4 or less*
___ Evaluation: _____ *during post-op recovery*

Nursing Intervention Standards:
1. Assess pain and related factors.
   a. intensity (1–10) *rated as 8 on admission*
   b. duration *continuous; previously lasted several hours*
   c. character (sharp, dull, shooting, burning) *sharp*
   d. location *Right Upper quadrant*
   e. precipitated by *unknown*

2. Assess for effectiveness of previous pain relief interventions
   a. previous medication (drug, dose, route, effectiveness on 1–10) ___
      ASA 10 gr taken at home "not helpful at all, made
   b. other helpful measures: __—__   *me nauseated"*

3. Offer *Demerol 50-100 mg* (analgesic ordered by MD) q *3-4 h* prn.   *IM*
   6/6 Post-op Demerol 75-100 mg IM
4. Encourage use of analgesics before *tests*
   (pain precipitating activity) at _____ am/pm or _____

5. Offer relaxation techniques: slow relaxed breathing *explained 6/3*
                                music __—__
                                backrub *q h s*
                                heat __—__

6. Assist with repositioning as needed q *4° position of comfort*
   6/6 assist q 2° c̄ repositioning
7. Encourage use of distracting stimuli: radio, (TV) other: _____
   effleurage/skin stroking *RUQ by patient ad lib*
   6/6 disc. eff.

Developed by *L. Atkinson RN*   date: *6/3/90*
Evaluated by *L. Atkinson RN*   date: *6/3/90*
Reviewed/Updated by *L. Atkinson RN*   date: *6/6/90*

Bibliography

AMERICAN NURSE'S ASSOCIATION (1973). *Standards for Nursing Practice.* Kansas City, MO, American Nurses' Association, #NP.41.

ATKINSON, L.D., and MURRAY, M.E. (1985). *Fundamentals of Nursing: A Nursing Process Approach,* New York, Macmillan.

BRUNNER, L.S., and SUDDARTH, D.S. (1988). *Textbook of Medical-Surgical Nursing* (6th ed.). Philadelphia, Lippincott.

BULECHEK, G.M., and McCLOSKEY, J.C. (1989). Nursing Interventions: Treatments for Potential Nursing Diagnoses. In: Carroll-Johnson, R.M., (Ed.). (1989). *Classification of Nursing Diagnoses: Proceeding of the Eighth Conference.* North American Nursing Diagnosis Association, Philadelphia, Lippincott.

CARROLL-JOHNSON, R.M. (Ed.). (1989). *Classification of Nursing Diagnoses: Proceedings of the Eighth Conference.* North American Nursing Diagnosis Association, Philadelphia, Lippincott.

CARPENITO, L.J. (1989). *Handbook of Nursing Diagnosis.* Philadelphia, Lippincott.

CARPENITO, L.J. (1989). *Nursing Diagnosis: Application to Clinical Practice* (3rd ed.). Philadelphia, Lippincott.

FITZPATRICK, J.J., and WHALL, A.L. (1989). *Conceptual Models of Nursing: Analysis and Application* (2nd ed.). Norwalk, CT, Appleton & Lang.

GORDON, M. (1982). *Nursing Diagnosis.* New York, McGraw-Hill.

GORDON, M. (1982). *Nursing Diagnosis: Process and Application.* New York, McGraw-Hill.

HENDERSON, V. (1978). *The Nature of Nursing.* New York, Macmillan.

121

JOINT COMMISSION ON ACCREDITATION OF HEALTH CARE ORGANIZATIONS (1988). *AMH Accreditation Manual for Hospitals 1989.* Chicago.

LANG, N.M., and GEBBIE, K. (1989). Nursing Taxonomy: NANDA and ANA Joint Venture toward ICD-10CM. In: Carroll-Johnson, R.M., (Ed.). (1989). *Classification of Nursing Diagnoses: Proceedings of the Eighth Conference.* North American Nursing Diagnosis Association, Philadelphia, Lippincott.

LUCKMANN, J., and SORENSON, K.C. (1987). *Medical-Surgical Nursing* (3rd ed.). Philadelphia, Saunders.

MASLOW, A. (1968). *Toward a Psychology of Being.* New York, Van Nostrand.

NIGHTINGALE, F. (1969). *Notes on Nursing: What It Is and What It Is Not.* New York, Dover. (Originally published 1859).

TRIPP, S., and STACHOWIAK, B. (1989) Nursing diagnosis: health seeking behaviors (specify). In: Carroll-Johnson, R.M., (Ed.). (1989). *Classification of Nursing Diagnoses: Proceedings of the Eighth Conference.* North American Nursing Diagnosis Association, Philadelphia, Lippincott.

YURA, H., and WALSH, M.B. (1988). *The Nursing Process.* (5th ed.). Norwalk, CT, Appleton & Lange.

Sample Nursing Care Plans

STANDARD PLANS OF CARE

NURSING CARE PLAN #1. MIDDLE ADULT

Lyman, John
66550250
Dr. Burns/Snyder
Room 231 55 yrs

NURSING ASSESSMENT

(Data Collection Format based on the Functional Health Patterns developed by Gordon, 1982)

General Information

Information given by: patient

Name: Mr. John Lyman

Age: 55 yrs   Sex: male   Race: Caucasian

Admission date/time: 7/6/90; 2100 hours

Admitting medical diagnosis: "possible heart attack"

Arrived on unit by: wheelchair   from: home

Accompanied by: daughter

Admitting Weight/VS: T. 99.0, P. 96, R. 28, BP 120/70 ; 188 lbs, 5'11'

Allergies: no known allergies

Medications: no prescription meds

Health Perception-Health Management

Patient's Perception of Reason for Admission: severe pain in middle of chest, upper abdomen region; "The doctor thinks I might have had a heart attack;" "I've never had anything like this before."

How has problem been managed by patient at home? "I sat down and tried to relax, then I lay down but nothing helped; the chest pain just kept getting worse so I called the doctor and she said to come right in."

MIDDLE ADULT

Nutritional-Metabolic Pattern
states he is about 15 lbs overweight; eats 2–3 meals a day often skips breakfast; cooks for himself but eats out frequently; reports alcohol consumption of 2–3 drinks/week
Skin: mucous membranes pink; good skin turgor; diaphoretic, pale
Last intake: at 6 P.M. was a pizza; denies any nausea on admission
Food Allergies: none

Elimination Pattern
Bowel: last BM on 7/6; usual pattern qd; denies taking laxatives/softeners; bowel sounds present in all 4 quadrants
Urinary: denies any changes in urinary elimination patterns: no difficulty initiating; voids in large amounts, no burning; last voiding on admission to hospital—states it was normal large amount
Edema: no edema noted in ankles or fingers; denies any problem with edema; ring is not tight

Activity-Exercise Pattern
no physical limitations; reports going to the health club 2–3 times a week for weight machines and occasional racquetball games; no daily exercise program
Respiratory: reports slight dyspnea; some diaphoresis noted; respirations nonlabored but slightly deeper and more rapid than normal; lung sounds clear; no cyanosis noted on admission; smokes 2 packs/day; reports he has tried to quit twice but he really enjoys smoking and he lives alone so no one complains
Cardiac: normal BP 150/90; 120/70 on admission; pulse rapid, strong radial pulse, 96/min and irregular; patient reports feeling occasional palpitations for last hour; monitor shows normal sinus rhythm, occasional PVC's (1–4/min) over 15 minutes since admission

Sleep-Rest Pattern
6 hours a night is normal pattern; denies use of sleeping medications

NURSING CARE PLAN #1 (Cont.)

Cognitive-Perceptual Pattern

Pain: states he was watching TV when the pain started in the mid-chest area; described as viselike and radiated down left arm; "pain got worse and worse over about an hour"; rated as "8" on 1–10 scale

Analgesics: states he has taken nothing for pain but really needs something now

Senses: denies any hearing, speech, or visual problems; states he probably needs glasses because things are getting blurry up as close as he used to hold them; denies any changes in sensation, no numbness of fingers/ toes

Orientation: oriented to time, place, and person; states he feels "just awful" and is afraid he is going to die

Self-Perception–Self-Concept Pattern

reports being afraid of dying or being a burden to his family; "my father died of a heart attack in his 50s" and "I have had high blood pressure and an elevated cholesterol for 3 years that I know of"; three married daughters; one lives in town and brought him in; divorced 4 years ago from his wife of 25 years; lives alone and states he is very independent; "couldn't live with my daughters and have them take care of me"; reports he works hard and long hours as a financial advisor; "my daughters have been after me to take it easier and take some time off but I just never seem to find the time."

Role-Relationship Pattern

lives alone since divorce 4 years ago; ex-wife out of state and does not want her notified of his condition; three married daughters; visits the one in town every few weeks and occasionally babysits his grandchildren

Sexuality-Reproductive Pattern

vasectomy 1969; reports no problems with sexual part of his life; "I've kind of been on hold since the divorce"; "I suppose I won't have to worry about that anymore though; if this is a heart attack I know sex is out for me."

MIDDLE ADULT

Coping-Stress Tolerance Pattern

"I guess I am under a lot of stress at work; the stockmarket is hard to predict but my clients expect me to always make a profit; sometimes I feel like everyone is pulling on me to do things for them"; "I'm going to have to make a few phone calls to work, how do I get an outside line?"

Value-Belief Pattern

Catholic; attends church every week; reports he would like to see his priest if he gets worse

NURSING CARE PLAN #1 (Cont.)

Priority Nursing Diagnoses

Goals

1. Fear related to possible myocardial infarction and risk of dying as manifested by own statements, elevated pulse

   Reduction in fear reported; identification of methods of coping with/reducing fear of MI/dying/reoccurance by disch.

   - statement of feeling less fearful in 1 hour
   - states understanding of tests, treatments prior to implementing
   - states understanding of risk factors in life-style and changes needed to reduce risk by discharge

2. Pain related to possible myocardial hypoxia as manifested by rating pain an "8," elevated pulse and diaphoresis

   Report of negligible pain by discharge
   - pain reported at a level of 3 or less within the next hour with the use of IV morphine
   - pain maintained at a level of 3 or less during the next 48 hours with analgesics

3. Potential decreased cardiac output related to inadequate pumping of the heart secondary to possible MI (myocardial infarction)

   Maintains adequate tissue perfusion during hospitalization
   - maintains clear lung sounds during next 48 hours
   - presence of strong peripheral pulses during next 48 hours
   - maintains heart rate between 70–100 with no cyanosis while hospitalized

Nursing Interventions

Rationale

1. a. assess understanding and teach prn before tests, tx., interventions

   a. provides baseline data from which to teach; begin at learner's level of understanding; knowing what to expect decreases fear

MIDDLE ADULT

Nursing Interventions	*Rationale*
b. offer opportunity to share fears, concerns q4h x 24h; reassure realistically; point out positive sign of patient status/functioning	b. identifying and discussing fears gives nurse a chance to understand and support without giving false reassurance; focus on positive gives encouragement and hope
c. encourage daughter to stay with patient or visit	c. presence of support people can decrease fear; safety/security
d. have pt/family write down their questions for the doctor or nurse	d. unanswered questions/confusion can cause concern; patients often forget to ask questions when MD or nurse in room
e. orient to room; all equipment	e. unfamiliar environment can cause anxiety/fear
f. offer to contact hospital chaplain anytime patient desires	f. meeting spiritual needs can decrease anxiety and give hope; opportunity to express concerns
g. assign consistent nursing personnel whenever possible: Adams, Grahm, Tran	g. development of trusting therapeutic relationship decreases fear
h. involve patient in planning own care; explain how pt can maximize medical and nursing treatment to promote recovery	h. gives patient sense of control which can decrease fear; promotes cooperation with treatments
i. when physical status stabilizes: ○ assess knowledge of heart disease and risk factors in pt's life ○ provide information as needed ○ work with patient on problem-solving ways to reduce risk factors and attain maximum recovery ○ discuss possibility of family conference involving daughters, doctor, nurses for discussion of life-style changes; medical management of condition; abilities, limitations, schedule for resumption of activities and work responsibilities	i. readiness to learn life-style changes begins with recovery phase of illness; input and support from all involved result in more realistic plan, increased commitment to plan

NURSING CARE PLAN #1 (Cont.)

Nursing Interventions	*Rationale*
2.a. assess knowledge of reason for pain and assessments; explain as needed to patient/family	a. teaching begins at the learner's level of understanding to be most effective; understanding cause of pain makes tx. more understandable
b. assess vital signs and pain; begin morphine IV per doctor's order ◦ respirations, pulse and BP qh ◦ level of consciousness qh ◦ notify MD if r > 14, BP > 100/70 ◦ assess and reassure during first 15 min of morphine administration ◦ side rail up during administration	b. provides baseline data from which response to treatment is judged ◦ morphine can depress respirations ◦ morphine causes vasodilation and possible hypotensive response ◦ morphine can cause euphoric state; dizziness or fainting can occur if patient tries to stand
c. oxygen per doctor's order; assess concentration, response q 1h	c. morphine may depress respirations; increasing amount of oxygen to heart tissue will help reduce pain
d. position in semi-fowler's position (head of bed up at 45 degrees)	d. generally more comfortable position if SOB; lowers diaphragm and increases lung expansion
e. explain and implement bedrest order; place urinal, phone, water within reach	e. decreases work load on heart and oxygen requirements; may decrease pain
f. environmental management to promote rest	f. noisy, bright room with many people talking and doing things interferes with ability to rest and produces added stress/anxiety
g. offer techniques to promote relaxation/pain management	g. decreased muscle tension reduces oxygen needs of muscles; distraction, imagery can reduce perception of pain and promote rest

MIDDLE ADULT

Nursing Interventions	*Rationale*
3. a. assess per doctor's order and report significant changes to physician in areas of: ◦ vital signs q1h ◦ urine volume q2h or q voiding ◦ skin temp/peripheral pulses ◦ lung sounds ◦ regularity of heartbeat	a. assessment data provides baseline for comparison of changes which may indicate changing patient condition and need for adjustment of nursing and medical treatment plan; —decreased urine output may indicate inadequate blood flow to kidney; dehydration ◦ deterioration in pumping action of heart can lead to dropping BP, increased or decreased heart rate, increase in PVCs; cold pale skin and weak or absent pulses in extremities; build-up of fluid in lungs with moist breath sounds developing
b. oxygen per doctors order; assess concentration, response q1h (explain "no smoking" rule)	b. increased oxygen content of inspired air provides more oxygen to all body tissues; oxygen promotes burning and smoking could cause a fire
c. assist with position changes q2h (head of bed up at 45 degrees)	c. alternating pressure areas will promote adequate circulation and oxygenation of weight bearing body tissues
d. explain and implement bedrest order; place urinal, phone, water within reach	d. decreases work load on heart and improves circulation to legs
e. accurate intake/output recordings and daily weights	e. dehydration can decrease the circulating blood volume resulting in decreased perfusion of periphery; excess fluid can cause accumulation in the lungs; maintenance of normal weight reflects adequate hydration and no fluid retention

NURSING CARE PLAN #1. Middle Adult
(demonstrates individualization
of pretyped form for dx of "Pain")

Lyman, John
66550250
Dr. Burns/Snyder
Room 231   55 yrs

Nursing Diagnosis Standard Care Plan: Pain

Pain related to *myocardial hypoxia 7/6/90*
("A state in which an individual experiences and reports the presence of severe
discomfort or an uncomfortable sensation," NANDA, 1989)
Patient Characteristics: *pain rated as "8" on admission, P 96,
R 28, diaphoretic*

Patient Goals/Outcome Standards:

✓ Verbalization that pain has been eliminated or decreased to a level of _3_
   on a scale of 1–10 by *1 hr with use of IV morphine drip*
                       during *next 48 hrs c̄ analgesics)*
___ Evaluation: _____
NA Reduction of agitated/restless behavior by _____ .
   Evaluation: _____

✓ Reduction in values of vital signs, (P) (R) BP, toward normal range
   by *4 hrs* .
___ Evaluation: _____

Other: *Report of negligible pain by discharge c̄ no*
___ Evaluation: _____ *analgesics)*

Nursing Intervention Standards:
✓ 1. Assess pain and related factors.
   a. intensity (1–10) *8 on adm   2100 hrs   7/6* .
   b. duration *1 hr while at home*
   c. character (sharp, dull, shooting, burning)*viselike; radiates L*
   d. location *midchest & down L arm* . *arm*
   e. precipitated by *unknown; no precipitating exercise/activit*

✓ 2. Assess for effectiveness of previous pain relief interventions
    a. previous medication (drug, dose, route, effectiveness on 1–10)
       denies any
    b. other helpful measures: *none; sitting & lying at home, not helpful.*

✓ 3. Offer IV *morphine sulfate* ʌ (analgesic ordered by MD) *continuous* prn. *drip*

NA 4. Encourage use of analgesics before _____ (pain precipitating activity) at _____ am/pm or _____

✓ 5. Offer relaxation techniques: slow relaxed breathing ✓; *relaxation*
    music __—__ heat __—__
    backrub ✓ *q 2h* other _____

✓ 6. Assist with repositioning (specify) *Semi-Fowlers* q *2 hrs*

✓ 7. Encourage use of distracting stimuli: radio, TV, effleurage, other: *imagery; quiet environment*

Developed by *L. atkinson RN*   date: *7/6/90*
Evaluated by _____ date: _____
Reviewed/Updated by _____ date: _____

NURSING CARE PLAN #2. SENIOR ADULT

Morgan, Fred
89645412
Dr. Sharp/Johnson
Room 109   78 years

NURSING ASSESSMENT

(Data Collection Format based on Human Response Patterns described by NANDA, 1989)

General Information
Information given by: patient and son
Name: Mr. Fred Morgan
Age: 78 yrs   Sex: male   Race: Caucasian
Admission date/time: 12/1/90; 2 P.M.
Admitting medical diagnosis: unable/unwilling to care for self at home; weight loss; mild hypertension history
Arrived on unit by: wheelchair   from: home
Accompanied by: son
Admitting Weight/VS: T. 97.0, P. 90, R. 20, BP 140/88; 154 lbs, 6'1"
Patient's Perception of Reason for Admission: "I don't need to be here. I'm just tired. I was fine when my wife was alive but now I don't get out much or do anything. My son's worried I don't eat."
How had problem been managed by patient at home? son visits every few weeks but says father is getting worse, isolated, losing weight
Allergies: no known allergies
Medications: "something for my blood pressure" (Inderal)

Exchanging
Nutrition: wears dentures, states they do not hurt; lips are pink but dry; poor skin turgor; appears gaunt, thin; reports normal smell but decreased taste to food; reports poor appetite; cooks for self; "Food just doesn't taste good any more"; son states father does not eat, won't shop for groceries; has lost 11 lbs in the last 2 months
Elimination: continent of bowel and bladder; denies taking laxatives; states normal pattern q.d.; denies trouble initiating or maintaining urination; voids large amounts several times a day

SENIOR ADULT

Circulation: heart rate 90 and regular; strong pulses; BP 140/88 on admission; son states it used to be higher and father put on medication several years ago; feet and hands pale, cool

Oxygenation: breath sounds clear; rate 20/minute; nonlabored; denies smoking; son says he quit 15 years ago; denies any difficulty breathing; son says lately his father tires easily and breathes harder with activity

Physical Integrity: skin intact, dry; mucous membranes intact, no open sores; son states father was not bathing, shaving, or doing personal hygiene; nails dirty

Communication

initiates no conversation; responds only to direct questions; denies any hearing problem; speech not impaired

Relating

Socialization: son states father used to be outgoing and was active with his wife in church and around the house; son states father has progressively withdrawn from contact and communication with friends/family since wife's death 6 months ago

Role: son states father was a carpenter but remained active with projects after retirement but now he doesn't do anything; doesn't call family or relate to grandchildren when visiting; patient states "I've got nothing to do; no point in doing anything anymore" denies having any close friends, "They are all dead or put away"; says son busy with his own life and doesn't have time for him (son lives out of town, 1 hour away; patients only child)

Valuing

states he used to go to church with his wife every Sunday but he did it for her so now there's no point going

Choosing

Coping: "I just don't care any more"; reports thinking about wife frequently. Son says his father is having trouble making even simple decisions so leaves bills, shopping, cooking, and so on unattended

NURSING CARE PLAN #2 (Cont.)

Moving
Mobility–Activity: son reports father tires more easily since he has lost weight, "stopped caring about himself"; no physical limitations; no activities except watching TV

Rest–Sleep: patient states tired all the time; can't sleep, wakes up 2–3 times/night; naps frequently; son states he is always sleeping in chair when he visits

Activities of Daily Living: son states he thinks father is able to live alone and manage for himself but just doesn't care anymore

Perceiving
Self-Concept: "states he is useless"; feels "helpless without his wife"; "no good to anyone any more"

Sensory–Perception: no changed sensations; wears bifocals; states he hears well

Knowing/Thought Processes
no evidence of altered thought processes; sentences logical, appropriate responses; oriented to time, place, and person

Feeling
Comfort: denies any pain; "stiff sometimes"

Emotional State/Integrity: crying occasionally during assessment; "I can't understand why she had to die. I wish it had been me. Its hard to be the one left." "I want to be with her again". Denies feeling suicidal, "I wouldn't do that."

SENIOR ADULT

Priority Nursing Diagnoses

1. Altered nutrition: less than body requirements related to lack of interest in food as manifested by 11 lb. weight loss over last 2 months.

2. Sleep pattern disturbance related to loss of wife, altered daytime activity pattern, frequent naps as evidenced by statements of inability to get to sleep, wakening 2–3 times per night, being tired all the time.

3. Dysfunctional grieving related to death of spouse as manifested by report of constantly thinking about his wife, crying, self-imposed social isolation, physical neglect of self.

4. Disturbance in self-esteem related to loss of spouse and husband role as manifested by statements of helplessness, uselessness, inability to do anything productive.

5. Potential for violence: self-directed related to negative self-esteem and depression as manifested by statements of wanting to be with dead wife, wishing it had been him that died.

Goals

1. Weight will stabilize at his previous level of 165 lbs within 3 months. Evaluate 5/1
   ○ weight gain of 3 lbs at the end of 2 weeks. Evaluate 2/15
   ○ report of appetite returning during the next week. Evaluate on 2/8

2. Sleeping 6 hours through the night during stay in nursing home.

3. Reestablishes previous level of self-care, productivity, social contacts by 3/1
   ○ expresses feelings related to loss of spouse within 1 week
   ○ identifies losses/changes in his life because of wife's death by 2nd week
   ○ identifies self-destructive or punishing behavior in self by 2 weeks
   ○ independently reestablishes previous level of personal grooming by 4 weeks

4. Evaluate self as needed and competent by 3 months
   ○ one positive statement of self-worth within 48 hours
   ○ begins work on one carpentry project by 2 weeks

5. Client will deny suicidal plans or ideas throughout stay in nursing home. Evaluate Fridays of each week.

NURSING CARE PLAN #2 (Cont.)

Nursing Interventions	*Rationale*
1. a. Observe, record, and report I & O.	1. a.b. Monitor client's progress/ evaluate effectiveness of plan.
b. Weigh q A.M.	
c. Assess food preferences.	c. Taking into account client's likes/dislikes may stimulate appetite.
d. Assist client in filling out daily menu.	d. Involve client in plan to increase cooperation. Ensure nutritionally balanced meal.
e. Consult with physician and dietitian regarding between-meal snacks, high calorie and high protein food supplements, possible vitamin supplements.	e. Meet nutritional needs of client.
f. Assist client with hygiene before meals.	f. Increase psychological and physical readiness to eat.
g. Encourage client to sit with others in the dining room @ mealtimes.	g. Normal eating situation tends to stimulate appetite.
2. a. Obtain a sleep history on pattern prior to death of wife and changes since death	2. a. Provides baseline data from which to assess activities that promote or interfere with sleep
b. Assess for factors in nursing home environment that might interfere with sleep and minimize if possible	b. Noise, heat, cold, too hard or soft a bed, roommates, lights, can all interfere with sleep
c. Increase daytime activity ∘ dining room for meals ∘ shower/bath daily; patient's choice ∘ walks on grounds/in building for 10–15 minutes QID ∘ encourage participation in group exercise sessions/ activities	c. Promotes normal circadian rhythm
d. Offer back rub at HS	d. Backrubs help to relax muscles and provide the patient time to talk about any concerns; relaxation and decreased anxiety facilitate sleep

Nursing Interventions	*Rationale*

e. Encourage good sleep hygiene
- no caffeine after noon meal
- limit cigarette smoking
- offer light snack before bed
- help to follow usual routine for hygiene, time to retire

e.
- caffeine is a stimulant
- nicotine can stimulate CNS
- foods high in protein and L-tryptophan (milk) promote sleep
- normal habits from home are associated with a good sleeping pattern

3. a. Assess the existence, extent and impact of unresolved losses through use of open-ended and direct questions.

3. a. Must assess types of unresolved losses and importance to client in order to fully implement plan (Note: elderly frequently have multiple unresolved losses).

b. Encourage client to verbalize feelings regarding losses.

b.c. Increase data base; assist client in developing an awareness of predominant feelings.

c. Share own observations of client's behavior and seek clarification/confirmation.

d. Spend 10 min sitting c̄ client b.i.d.; use touch as appropriate; remain c̄ client despite lack of ability to verbalize.

d. Build rapport, develop trust. Convey unconditional acceptance so client is free to express feelings.

e. Look over the daily activity calendar c̄ the client and leave a copy in his room; specifically suggest choosing one activity.

e. Involve client to improve co-operation. Individualize plan to insure its likelihood of success. Decrease isolation.

f. Encourage client to sit c̄ others in the dining room @ meal times.

f.g. Gradually "repeople" client's life; supply opportunities for development of meaningful interpersonal relationships s̄ overwhelming him. Reinforce sense of belonging.

g. Introduce client to other residents on the units.

4. a. Assess client's interests through use of open-ended and direct questions.

4. a. Necessary data to guide plan.

NURSING CARE PLAN #2 (Cont.)

Nursing Intervention	*Rationale*
b. Encourage patient to verbalize about himself, especially his present feelings.	b. Continue assessment. Convey acceptance of client. Increase client awareness of feelings.
c. Continue nursing actions 3.c. and 3.d.	c. Same as 3.c. and 3.d.
d. Maximize choices client can make.	d.e.f. Rebuild self-esteem.
e. Assist c̄ grooming as needed.	
f. Give merited praise and recognition based on specific, accurate observation.	
g. Occupational therapy referral for projects, needs of facility in carpentry.	g. projects useful to facility in field of expertise reinforce usefulness, positive self-worth.
5. a. Be direct in asking client if he is presently suicidal.	5. a. Determine immediate goal for intervention.
b. Make verbal agreement c̄ client that he will notify nursing staff if feeling out of control or suicidal.	b. Involve client in plan to ensure its success.
c. Move client to room closer to nurse's station if feeling suicidal.	c. Increase nurse's accessibility to client and increase opportunities for observation.
d. Increase frequency of room checks.	d. Prevent, interfere with, or interrupt any self-destructive behavior.
e. Monitor client behavior; observe especially for changes in mood/or levels of energy (be aware of greater risk following these changes).	e. Provide data c̄ which to evaluate suicide potential; changes may signal increased suicide risk.
f. Alert all staff regarding client's suicidal potential.	f. Provide safety and security for client.
g. Spend 10 min. sitting c̄ client b.i.d.; use touch as appropriate; remain c̄ client despite lack of verbalization.	g. Build rapport, develop trust. Convey unconditional acceptance so client is free to express feelings.
h. Permit verbalization of suicidal feelings, do not ignore them or argue c̄ client about them.	h. Establish trust. Recognize importance of intent.
i. Carefully document client behavior and nursing actions.	i. Ensure consistency of care.

NURSING CARE PLAN #2. Senior Adult
(demonstrates individualization
of pretyped form for dx of "Altered Nutrition")

Morgan, Fred
89645412
Dr. Sharp/Johnson
Room 109   78 yrs

Nursing Diagnosis Standard Care Plan: Altered Nutrition

Altered Nutrition: less than body requirements related to *lack of*
interest in food; progressively worse since wife's death
("The state in which an individual experiences an intake of nutrients insufficient
to meet metabolic needs," NANDA, 1989)
Patient Characteristics: *weight loss of 11 lbs in last 2 months;*
appears gaunt, dry skin, poor turgor, states
"Food just doesn't taste good anymore"

Patient Goals/Outcome Standards:
NA Maintains current weight by _____ for _____
Evaluation: _____

NA Tolerates diet of _____ by _____
Evaluation: _____

✓ Gains **3 lbs** _____ each day/week/month **every 2 wks** by *12/15*
Evaluation: _____

✓ Consumes _____ calories/day or **50% or more**% of meals by *12/3*
Evaluation: _____

✓ Identifies factors contributing to inadequate intake by *12/5*
Evaluation: _____

✓ Patient demonstrates ability to (plan)/(prepare) *2000 calorie*
diet to meet needs by *time of discharge if able to leave*
Evaluation: _____ *nursing home*

✓ Reports good appetite by *12/8*
Evaluation: _____

NURSING CARE PLAN #2 (Cont.)

✓ Regains lost weight of ____11____ lbs by __3/1/91__ ; maintains target weight of __165 oz ↑__ for _duration of stay in_
Evaluation: _____ _nursing home_

Other: _____
    Evaluation: _____

Nursing Intervention Standards:
  ✓1. Assess current dietary intake and related factors. _small supper_
     a. meals/snacks per day _snacks when hungry; eats Bkf &⁵_
     b. types of foods eaten _sandwiches, cereal, toast_
     c. changes in eating patterns _wife used to cook all meals- B,L,D_
     d. factors interfering with adequate intake (physical,) (psychological,) financial, (educational) _↓appetite; ↓ sense of taste, no groceries in home, doesn't like to shop or cook for self_
     e. favorite foods/fluids _wife's cooking; meat & potatoes_
     f. help needed with eating _none; enc. to eat_
  ✓2. Assist with meals by _enc. out of bed & to dining room; enc. to eat at least ½ of each food on tray; praise_
  ✓3. Problem-solve with patient/family on ways to reduce factors interfering with adequate diet.
     Discharge planning should include senior meals program delivered to home
  ✓4. Referral to (dietary) social service/public health nurse/other _physician for any diet restrictions related to hypertension_
  ✓5. Record I&O; encourage (patient) family participation in recording.
  ✓6. Offer opportunity for (patient) family to talk about reasons for not eating _q od at H.S._ .
  ✓7. Encourage smaller meals; _choc. shake_ in between snacks; favorite foods
  ✓8. Adapt environmental factors to promote appetite/eating _open curtains; time for cleaning dentures & out of bed b/4 meals_
  ✓9. Weigh: _q d & record_
  ✓10. Good oral hygiene before and after meals. self _✓ enc._ assist ____
  ✓11. Promote socialization during meals by: _intro to other residents in dining room._
  ✓12. Other interventions: _Discuss relationship between grief & depression; effect on appetite; food consumption_

Developed by _L. atkinson RN 12/1/90_

Index